EARLY PERIMENOPAUSE MASTERY

Reclaim Your Identity_ Preserve Your
Career and Predict Symptom Patterns
Without Medical Dismissal

Lily Wright

Anthony Fallon Publishing

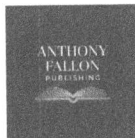

ISBN:978-1-0682005-9-5 eBook
ISBN: 978-1-0682248-0-5 Paperback
ISBN: 978-1-0682248-1-2 HardBack

Cover design by: AFP
A CIP Catalogue record for this book is available from the British Library
Printed in the United States of America

CONTENTS

INTRODUCTION: THE PREMATURE TRANSITION PARADOX

---

*Your body whispers a truth your
mind refuses to accept.*

The symptoms appear without warning—night sweats that drench your sheets while you're only 37, brain fog that makes you forget your presentation points mid-meeting, mood shifts that leave you crying in your office bathroom. These physical realities clash violently with your mental image of yourself: a capable, professional woman in her prime. The disconnect is jarring, almost impossible to reconcile.

This is the premature transition paradox.

The Blindsiding Reality of Early Symptoms

Sarah, a 38-year-old marketing director, sat in her car before an executive presentation, frantically dabbing at sweat stains forming under her blazer. The air conditioning blasted at full power despite the cool autumn morning. For months, these sudden heat surges had ambushed her at the worst possible moments—during client pitches, board meetings, and her daughter's parent-teacher conferences. Her doctor had dismissed her concerns with a casual, "You're much too young for menopause. It's probably stress from your busy job."

But Sarah knew her body. This wasn't normal workplace pressure. The night sweats, waking her at 3 AM, weren't explained by her project deadlines. The memory lapses —forgetting words mid-sentence during presentations she'd prepared for weeks—weren't just "mommy brain" as her physician suggested with a patronising smile. Something fundamental was changing, and nobody seemed to have answers that matched her experience.

Sarah's story reflects a reality faced by thousands of professional women between the ages of 35 and 45. You might recognise elements of your own experience in hers—the confusion, the medical dismissal, the desperate search for explanations that align with how you're feeling rather than how others think you should feel based on your age.

What Sarah was experiencing—what you may be experiencing —has a name: early perimenopause. This transition phase before menopause can begin in your 30s, despite medical textbooks and cultural narratives suggesting it's a decade or more away. The physical symptoms alone are challenging enough, but the psychological impact of facing this transition "too early" creates a unique burden that conventional resources fail to address.

Early perimenopause isn't just about physical symptoms—it's about a profound identity disruption that occurs when your biological reality contradicts your chronological self-concept.

The Isolation of Being Decades "Too Early"

"Have you considered that it might be anxiety?" the third doctor asked Michelle, a 41-year-old financial analyst who'd been tracking her increasingly irregular periods, insomnia, and concentration problems for eight months. She left the appointment with yet another recommendation for stress management techniques and a thinly veiled suggestion that perhaps she should consider scaling back her "ambitious" career goals.

The medical dismissal was frustrating, but equally difficult was the isolation. Her friends, most of whom were also in their early 40s, couldn't relate to her experiences. Online forums and support groups were dominated by women in their 50s discussing symptoms that had begun at "appropriate" ages. Books and articles about perimenopause seemed to address a different demographic entirely—women whose children were grown, whose careers were established, whose identities had already shifted toward middle age.

Michelle found herself in a no-woman 's land, experiencing significant hormonal changes without the validation, support, or guidance available to women entering this transition a decade later.

This isolation isn't accidental. It stems from deeply entrenched misconceptions about women's health transitions:

Common Misconception	Biological Reality
Perimenopause begins in your late 40s or early 50s.	Hormonal fluctuations can start in your mid-30s.
Symptoms appear in a predictable sequence.	Early perimenopause often presents with cognitive symptoms first.
You'll know it when it happens.	Many symptoms mimic stress, depression, or thyroid issues.
Medical tests can diagnose	Standard hormone tests

perimenopause.	often fail to detect early fluctuations in hormone levels.
Resources exist for all women in transition.	Most resources target women 10+ years older.

When you're experiencing something society insists shouldn't be happening to you, yet the psychological impact goes beyond the physical symptoms themselves. You may question your perceptions, wonder if you're overreacting, or blame yourself for not managing stress better. This self-doubt compounds the isolation, creating a cycle that deepens your sense of dislocation.

You are not alone in this experience. Your symptoms are not imaginary. Your timeline is not "wrong." The problem isn't your perception—it's the limited understanding of women's health transitions that fails to acknowledge the spectrum of everyday experiences.

The Chronological-Biological Identity Clash

At 36, Elena couldn't reconcile the woman she saw in the mirror—energetic, career-focused, mother of a toddler—with the biological signals her body was sending. The cognitive symptoms hit hardest: struggling to find words in meetings, forgetting important details, and losing her train of thought mid-conversation. As a professor who prided herself on intellectual sharpness, these changes struck at the core of her identity.

"I feel like my body is ageing faster than my life," she confided to her therapist. "I'm still building my career. My son just started preschool. My friends are talking about having their first babies, and my body is moving into a phase associated with my mother's generation. Who am I supposed to be right now?"

Elena's question gets to the heart of the premature transition paradox. When your biological experience contradicts your chronological identity—the sense of self associated with your actual age and life stage—it creates profound cognitive dissonance. This isn't just about physical discomfort; it's about your fundamental sense of who you are and where you belong in the trajectory of your own life.

This identity disruption manifests in several ways:

1. **Professional identity threats**: When brain fog, memory issues, and emotional regulation challenges impact your performance at work during critical career-building years

2. **Relational dissonance**: When symptoms affect your partnerships, parenting, and social connections in ways that feel premature or misaligned with your life stage

3. **Temporal displacement**: When you're forced to confront biological realities typically associated with a later life phase while still navigating early- or mid-adulthood challenges

4. **Narrative disruption**: When your life story no longer follows the expected timeline, requiring integration of an unexpected chapter

The conventional wisdom surrounding perimenopause—that it represents a natural "winding down" process, aligning with children leaving home and career peaks already achieved—doesn't serve the early transitioner. Your transition is happening alongside career advancement, active parenting, and other midlife building phases, not after them.

This timing creates unique challenges that require specific strategies—not just for managing symptoms, but for preserving and protecting your core identity during this unexpected transition.

The Transformative Promise: Identity Preservation Through Protocol Mastery

The standard approach to perimenopause management fails the early transitioner in two critical ways. First, it typically begins with acceptance, surrendering to the idea that this is simply a natural part of the ageing process. Second, it focuses primarily on symptom relief rather than identity preservation.

For a woman in her 50s whose career is established and whose children are grown, this approach might be sufficient. For you, in your prime working years, possibly raising young children, still building toward life goals, simple symptom management isn't enough. You need strategies that protect your professional trajectory, maintain your cognitive function, preserve your relationships, and sustain your core identity while you navigate this transition.

This book offers a fundamentally different approach. Rather than asking you to accept these changes or surrender aspects of your identity passively, it provides a structured framework for:

1. **Maintaining your core identity** throughout the transition

2. **Mastering specific protocols** that transform unpredictable symptoms into manageable patterns

3. **Integrating biological changes** without surrendering your chronological self-concept

4. **Protecting your professional performance** during cognitive fluctuations

5. **Preserving key relationships** through strategic communication

The transformative promise is this: You can navigate early perimenopause without losing yourself in the process. Your symptoms don't have to derail your career, damage your relationships, or diminish your sense of self. With the right approach, you can integrate this unexpected biological reality while maintaining the core elements of who you are and what matters most to you.

This isn't about denying reality or fighting against natural processes. It's about managing this transition on your terms, with strategies specifically designed for your unique circumstances as an early transitioner.

The BICEP Framework: Your Structured Solution

The key insight that transforms the early perimenopause experience is this: Early transition thrives through structured protocols, not passive acceptance. Random approaches yield random results. Structured protocols transform chaos into manageable processes.

The BICEP Framework provides that structure. This systematic approach addresses both symptom management and identity preservation through five integrated steps:

B - Baseline: Establishing your symptom patterns, identity markers, and life priorities to create a strong foundation for managing this transition

I - Intervention: Implementing targeted protocols matched to your specific symptom clusters and timed according to your unique hormonal patterns

C - Communication: Developing effective dialogue strategies for medical providers, partners, colleagues, and family members to maintain critical relationships during this transition

E - Evaluation: Tracking progress and refining your approach based on measurable results rather than subjective impressions

P - Projection: Creating a forward-focused identity that integrates your transitional wisdom while maintaining core self-elements

Unlike general wellness advice that might work for anyone at any life stage, these protocols are specifically designed for women experiencing perimenopause during peak career and family years. They address the unique challenges of managing cognitive symptoms in professional settings, navigating relationship changes while raising children, and preserving your sense of self when facing premature ageing signals.

Throughout this book, you'll learn how to implement each component of the framework in practical, manageable ways that respect your limited time and energy. You'll develop personalised protocols that address your specific symptom patterns rather than generic approaches that may or may not work for your unique situation.

The BICEP Framework transforms your relationship with early perimenopause from one of helpless victim to strategic navigator. It puts you back in control, not by denying reality, but by giving you practical tools to manage it.

The Journey Ahead

In the pages that follow, we'll explore each aspect of the premature transition paradox in detail. Part I focuses on recognition—understanding the biological reality of early perimenopause, the identity challenges it creates, the patterns hidden within seemingly chaotic symptoms, and the advocacy strategies needed to secure appropriate medical care.

Part II guides you through integration—implementing the BICEP Framework step by step to reconcile your chronological identity with your biological experience. You'll learn specific protocols for establishing baselines, implementing targeted interventions, communicating effectively with others, evaluating your progress, and projecting a positive future identity.

Part III takes you to mastery—refining your protocols for advanced symptom management, preserving your career during fluctuations, evolving your relationships, partnering effectively with medical providers, navigating crises, integrating your identity in the long term, and potentially contributing to a broader understanding of early perimenopause.

Throughout this journey, you'll meet women like Sarah, Michelle, and Elena—early transitioners who have successfully navigated this unexpected chapter without surrendering their core identities or derailing their life trajectories. Their stories will show you what's possible when you approach this transition with the right tools and strategies.

Your perimenopause may have started earlier than expected, but your response to it doesn't have to be left to chance. With structured protocols rather than passive acceptance, you can transform this challenging transition into an integrated part of your life story—one that doesn't diminish who you are but potentially enriches it.

As we move into Chapter 1, we'll begin by examining why your body isn't lying to you—even when medical providers, friends, or family members suggest otherwise. We'll look at the biological reality of hormonal transitions beginning in your 30s and why these changes are so frequently missed or dismissed by healthcare systems.

CHAPTER 1. YOUR BODY ISN'T LYING

---

*Your body sends signals long before
your brain can name them.*

These signals—night sweats that wake you at 3 AM, brain fog during critical meetings, mood swings that seem to come from nowhere—speak a truth your medical providers might dismiss, and your friends might misunderstand. What makes these experiences so unsettling isn't just their physical impact, but the profound confusion they create when you're told they shouldn't be happening "at your age." Your body isn't malfunctioning or overreacting—it's experiencing a legitimate biological transition.

Distinguishing Early Signs from Everyday Stressors

Sarah, a 37-year-old marketing executive, tracked her symptoms for months before our first meeting. "My doctor kept saying it was burnout," she explained, showing me meticulous notes documenting sleep disruptions, concentration lapses, and unpredictable mood shifts. "But I've been stressed before. This feels fundamentally different."

Sarah's experience highlights a common challenge: the substantial overlap between perimenopause symptoms and other conditions. Her doctor's diagnosis seemed logical: a high-powered executive with young children experiencing fatigue, anxiety, and concentration problems must be burning out, right?

Wrong. While stress and hormonal transitions can create similar symptoms, several key differences exist:

Perimenopause Indicators	Stress/Burnout Indicators
Symptoms follow cyclical patterns.	Symptoms directly correlate with stressful events.
Night sweats and hot flashes, especially at night.	General sleep disruption without temperature changes.
Physical symptoms persist despite stress management.	Symptoms improve with rest and stress reduction.
Menstrual cycle changes (heavier, lighter, irregular).	Minimal impact on the menstrual cycle.
Symptoms worsen at specific cycle points.	Consistent symptom intensity regardless of cycle timing.

The distinction lies not just in what you experience but in the patterns these experiences follow. Early perimenopause symptoms often:

- Fluctuate predictably with hormonal shifts
- Include distinct physical manifestations (temperature changes, menstrual irregularities)
- Respond differently to interventions than stress-related symptoms
- Create a sense of "body betrayal" that feels qualitatively different from exhaustion

The key differentiator is pattern recognition. When you track your symptoms alongside your menstrual cycle (even when it seems regular), connections often emerge that wouldn't align with purely stress-driven issues.

Laura, a 39-year-old attorney, noticed her brain fog consistently peaked 3-4 days before her period started—a pattern that remained stable even when her work stress fluctuated dramatically. "That consistency was my first clue," she explained. "Bad weeks at work made everything worse, but the cognitive symptoms followed a hormonal timeline, not my case schedule."

The Biological Reality of Early Transitions

Medical textbooks traditionally place perimenopause between the ages of 45 and 55, creating a blind spot for women experiencing symptoms earlier. However, current research shows hormonal changes begin much sooner than previously recognised:

1. **Reproductive ageing starts in your 30s**. Follicle-stimulating hormone (FSH) levels begin rising and anti-Müllerian hormone (AMH) levels start declining years before noticeable cycle changes.

2. **Hormonal fluctuations precede cycle changes**. Your periods might remain regular while hormones fluctuate wildly behind the scenes, creating symptoms without apparent menstrual irregularity.

3. **The transition occurs over years, not months**. The conventional perspective of menopause as a singular event misrepresents what's a decade-long process that can begin in your mid-30s.

Recent large-scale studies and surveys provide strong evidence that a significant proportion of women as young as 30–35 report moderate to severe perimenopausal or menopause-related symptoms, based on self-reported data using the Menopause Rating Scale (MRS):

A 2025 study published in _NJP Women's Health_ analysed

responses from over 4,400 American women aged 30 and older, collected via an online survey and the Flo app. Among women aged 30–35, 55.4% reported symptoms classified as "moderate" or "severe" on the MRS

The study emphasised that these findings are based on self-reported symptoms, not on longitudinal tracking of hormonal markers. The authors acknowledged that while some symptoms (such as mood changes) may have alternative explanations, the high rate of moderate to severe symptoms in younger women warrants further investigation.

Many women in this age group mistakenly believe they are too young to be affected by perimenopause, leading to delayed treatment and prolonged discomfort. The average age at which women seek treatment for menopause-associated symptoms was reported to be 56 or older, indicating a substantial delay between symptom onset and medical attention. These findings align with what many clinicians who specialise in women's hormonal health have observed for years—the transition timeline varies dramatically between individuals, with some women entering perimenopause a decade earlier than population averages suggest.

Jessica, a 36-year-old teacher, brought lab results to our second meeting. "My doctor finally ran hormone panels when I insisted," she said. "My FSH was elevated, and my Estrogen was all over the place. She was surprised, but I wasn't."

Jessica's experience highlights an essential truth: population averages create dangerous blind spots for individual women. The statistical "norm" of perimenopause at 45+ becomes a barrier to proper diagnosis when you fall outside that range.

Why Medical Dismissal Happens

Medical providers miss early perimenopause for several interconnected reasons:

Age-based diagnostic assumptions create an immediate barrier to effective treatment. When a 38-year-old reports night sweats, brain fog, and mood changes, many providers automatically look to stress, depression, or thyroid issues rather than hormonal transitions. This presumptive diagnosis often persists even when those conditions are ruled out.

Limited training in women's midlife health doesn't help the problem. A lot of medical education dedicates minimal time to perimenopause, focusing instead on pregnancy and post-menopausal conditions. This gap leaves many unprepared to recognise early transition symptoms.

Fluctuating lab results further complicate diagnosis. Unlike menopause (defined by 12 months without periods), perimenopause lacks definitive diagnostic tests. Hormone levels fluctuate dramatically, and blood tests often capture only a moment in time, missing the pattern of hormonal chaos that defines this transition.

Rachel, a 41-year-old finance professional, consulted with three doctors before finding one who recognised her symptoms. "Each one ran the same basic tests and told me I was fine when they came back 'normal.' But they were testing on different days of my cycle, getting completely different results, and never connecting the dots."

The diagnostic obstacles extend beyond individual provider limitations to systemic issues:

- Electronic health record templates rarely include perimenopause as a diagnosis option for women under 45

- Insurance coding requirements may not support perimenopause treatment in younger women

- Treatment protocols often focus on managing isolated symptoms rather than addressing the hormonal foundation

- Time constraints in standard appointments limit thorough symptom exploration

These structural barriers create a perfect storm of dismissal, leaving you to question your perceptions when your symptoms don't align with the expected timeline.

Early Warning Signs You Shouldn't Ignore

While every woman's perimenopause experience differs, specific patterns suggest hormonal shifts rather than other conditions:

Cognitive changes often appear before physical symptoms, including:

- Word-finding difficulties during presentations or meetings
- Short-term memory lapses that feel different from normal forgetfulness
- Difficulty maintaining focus on complex tasks that previously came easily

Sleep disruptions with specific characteristics:

- Waking between 2-4 AM, often with a racing heart or feeling overheated
- Difficulty returning to sleep after waking
- Sleep quality changes predictably at specific points in your cycle

Mood shifts with timing patterns:

- Increased anxiety or irritability that follows cyclical patterns
- Emotional reactions disproportionate to triggers
- Mood changes that cluster around specific cycle days

Physical indicators beyond menstrual changes:

- Temperature regulation issues (particularly at night or in controlled environments)

- Joint pain that migrates or fluctuates without an apparent cause

- Heart palpitations or racing pulse without cardiac issues

The appearance of even a few of these symptoms, especially when they follow cyclical patterns, warrants further investigation regardless of your age.

Moving Forward with Clarity

Recognising early perimenopause isn't about accepting a label—it's about validating your experience and creating a foundation for effective management. When you understand what's happening in your body, you can:

1. **Trust your perceptions**. Your symptoms aren't imaginary, exaggerated, or "just stress."

2. **Recognise patterns**. What seems random often follows predictable hormonal fluctuations that you can track, predict, and manage.

3. **Seek appropriate care**. With proper knowledge, you can advocate effectively within the medical system rather than accepting dismissal.

4. **Implement targeted strategies**. General wellness advice isn't enough—your symptoms require specific approaches designed for hormonal transitions.

The validation that comes from recognising early perimenopause isn't merely emotional comfort; it's the necessary first step toward regaining control. You cannot effectively manage what you don't understand, and you cannot advocate for appropriate care when doubting your own experience.

In the coming chapters, we'll build on this foundation of recognition to develop systematic approaches for managing your transition. Understanding that your body isn't lying is just the beginning—the fundamental transformation comes from turning that understanding into action through structured protocols that help preserve your identity during this unexpected biological shift.

Next, we'll explore how to maintain your core identity, addressing the psychological impact of premature ageing signals and develop strategies to protect the essential elements of how you see yourself in the world.

CHAPTER 2. IDENTITY IN TRANSITION

---

*Your body changes at thirty-eight, but
your self-concept refuses to follow.*

This disconnect creates one of the most challenging aspects of early perimenopause: reconciling who you believe yourself to be with what your body is experiencing. For women in their late thirties and early forties, this cognitive dissonance typically occurs during a life phase associated with peak performance and capability, rather than hormonal fluctuations. The psychological toll of this mismatch extends far beyond physical symptoms, creating a profound identity crisis that requires strategic navigation.

The Psychological Impact of Premature Biological Ageing Signals

Claire, a 39-year-old marketing executive, first noticed her memory lapses during a high-stakes presentation. "I suddenly couldn't remember our newest client's name—information I'd reviewed just minutes earlier. In that moment, I felt like someone else had inhabited my body. Who was this person who couldn't recall basic facts?"

This experience illustrates how early perimenopause creates a jarring collision between biological reality and psychological self-perception. When your body sends signals typically associated with women 10-15 years older, the disconnection triggers psychological distress that goes beyond mere symptom management.

This premature ageing process creates several psychological challenges:

- **Identity discontinuity** - The sudden shift disrupts your sense of a continuous, coherent self
- **Time compression** - Life transitions you expected decades later arrive prematurely
- **Social role confusion** - You may feel caught between peer groups, belonging neither with same-age friends nor with older women experiencing similar symptoms

*Research from the Institute of Women's Health shows that women experiencing perimenopause before age 45 report significantly higher rates of psychological distress compared to women experiencing symptoms at more expected ages. This isn't merely about discomfort with symptoms—it reflects a profound challenge to your fundamental sense of self.

Why Cognitive Symptoms Create the Deepest Identity Threat for Professionals

Not all perimenopause symptoms challenge your identity equally. For professional women, cognitive symptoms create particularly profound threats to self-concept.

Consider this comparison of symptom impact on professional identity:

Symptom Type	Example	Identity Impact
Physical	Hot flashes, night sweats	Moderate - primarily embarrassment or discomfort

Emotional	Mood swings, irritability	Significant - challenges the sense of emotional regulation
Cognitive	Brain fog, memory issues, word-finding difficulties	Severe - directly threatens core competence identity

Dr. Rebecca Thompson, a neuropsychologist specialising in hormonal cognitive changes, explains: "For professional women, cognitive abilities form a cornerstone of self-worth. When these capacities fluctuate unexpectedly, the effect goes beyond practical challenges to strike at fundamental beliefs about who you are."

Sarah, a 41-year-old attorney, describes this experience: "I built my career on quick thinking and verbal agility. When I started struggling to find words during court appearances, I questioned everything about myself. Hot flashes were annoying, but they didn't make me wonder if I could still do my job."

A 2023 study of professional women experiencing early perimenopause supports Sarah's experience. For professionals, these cognitive challenges arrive precisely when career demands are often highest:

- Mid-career advancement opportunities requiring peak performance
- Leadership roles with significant decision-making responsibility
- Periods of maximum earning potential
- Complex family obligations requiring executive function

- Little established flexibility for "off days"

This creates a perfect storm where identity threat coincides with high performance expectations, amplifying both practical challenges and psychological distress.

Distinguishing Between Your Chronological Self and Biological Processes

Michelle, a 37-year-old tech executive, initially panicked when perimenopause symptoms began. "I thought, 'Is this who I am now? A middle-aged woman who can't remember things and gets hot flashes in meetings?" After working with a therapist specialising in women's health transitions, Michelle gained a different perspective: "I learned to see these as biological processes happening to my body, not fundamental changes to who I am."

This distinction—separating biological processes from core identity—creates the foundation for psychological resilience during early perimenopause.

The Biological-Process-vs-Identity Framework helps establish this separation:

Biological processes:

- Hormonal fluctuations
- Resulting symptoms
- Physical responses
- Temporary capacity changes

Core identity elements:

- Professional capabilities and knowledge
- Key personal values
- Relationship roles
- Essential character traits

· Long-term goals and aspirations

By making this distinction, you create psychological space between "what's happening to my body" and "who I am as a person." This separation doesn't deny the reality of symptoms or their impact—it simply prevents them from defining your entire self-concept.

Laura Evans, a psychotherapist, counsellor, and CBT therapist in the UK, recommends a regular self-check using the following question: "If these symptoms disappeared tomorrow, what core aspects of myself would remain unchanged?" This exercise helps reinforce the distinction between temporary biological states and enduring aspects of identity.

Common Identity Preservation Mistakes That Increase Distress

Many women inadvertently amplify psychological distress through counterproductive responses to early perimenopause. These familiar patterns can undermine identity preservation efforts:

1. Total symptom denial

Kathryn, a 40-year-old financial analyst, ignored escalating symptoms for nearly a year. "I convinced myself it was just stress or lack of sleep. Admitting perimenopause meant accepting I was ageing, and I wasn't ready for that." This denial prevented her from implementing management strategies, allowing symptoms to worsen and eventually forcing a more dramatic identity reckoning.

2. Premature identity surrender

On the opposite end, some women abandon their established identity too quickly. Jennifer, a 39-year-old teacher, explains: "The moment I realised these were perimenopause symptoms, I started thinking of myself as 'old' and incapable. I withdrew from professional development opportunities and stopped applying for leadership positions." This premature surrender of identity created unnecessary limitations based on assumptions rather than actual capacity changes.

3. Binary thinking

Many women fall into an all-or-nothing trap regarding their capabilities. "Either I can perform exactly as I always have, or I'm completely incompetent," explains Laura Evans. "This binary thinking creates enormous pressure and fails to accommodate the normal fluctuations that perimenopause involves."

4. Catastrophic projection

"I'll never be able to function normally again" represents the kind of catastrophic thinking that amplifies distress. This future-focused anxiety creates psychological suffering beyond the actual symptom impact and makes objective assessment impossible.

5. Over-identification with symptoms

When symptoms become the central focus of your attention and conversation, they can gradually consume your self-concept. This over-identification can transform temporary experiences into defining characteristics, reinforcing rather than challenging their impact on identity.

The Balanced Approach:

Rather than these extremes, a balanced approach acknowledges fundamental biological changes while protecting core identity elements. This means:

- Recognising and addressing symptoms without allowing them to define you

- Adapting strategies while maintaining commitment to core goals

- Accommodating fluctuations without assuming permanent limitations

- Distinguishing between temporary symptoms and permanent transitions

Mapping Core Identity Elements That Require Active Protection

Not all aspects of identity require equal protection during perimenopause. The Identity Anchor Inventory helps you identify your most essential self-concept elements—those worth investing significant effort to preserve.

To create your Identity Anchor Inventory, consider these categories:

Professional identity elements:

- Specific expertise or skills central to your work
- Professional values you're unwilling to compromise
- Career trajectory elements are most essential to maintain
- Workplace relationships are crucial to your professional satisfaction

Relationship identity elements:

- Key roles in significant relationships (partner, parent, friend)
- Ways of being in relationships that feel essential to your self-concept
- Types of connection you're unwilling to surrender
- Relationship patterns you wish to maintain despite symptom challenges

Personal identity elements:

- Character traits you consider fundamental to who you are
- Values that guide your most important decisions

- Activities that contribute significantly to your sense of self
- Longer-term goals that shape your sense of purpose and direction

Once you've identified these elements, prioritise them based on:

1. Importance to your core self-concept
2. Level of threat from current or anticipated symptoms
3. Practical feasibility of protection strategies

This prioritisation ensures that you focus your limited energy on preserving what matters most to your sense of self.

Case Study: Identity Preservation in Action

Lisa, a 42-year-old university professor, created her Identity Anchor Inventory when cognitive symptoms began affecting her work. She identified teaching excellence and research contributions as her most essential elements of professional identity, while committee service ranked lower. This clarity allowed her to strategically reallocate her energy, protecting her most identity-relevant activities while finding ways to reduce commitments in less central areas temporarily.

"I couldn't do everything exactly as before," Lisa explains. "But by identifying what truly constituted my core professional identity, I could focus my best hours on those elements. This selective approach preserved what mattered most while I developed symptom management strategies."

This strategic approach—identifying what matters most and focusing protection efforts there—creates sustainable continuity of identity, even when adaptations become necessary in other areas.

Integrating Biological Reality With Chronological Identity

Your goal isn't to deny biological changes or cling rigidly to an unchanged identity. Instead, aim for strategic integration that accommodates new realities while preserving your fundamental sense of self.

This integration process involves:

1. Acknowledgement without surrender - Recognise biological changes without allowing them to override your entire self-concept

2. Strategic adaptation - Develop specific approaches to maintaining key identity elements despite symptom challenges

3. Narrative continuity - Create a coherent story that incorporates this unexpected transition while maintaining your sense of a continuous self

4. Selective flexibility - Identify areas where adaptation creates less identity threat and focus flexibility there

5. Future self-projection - Develop a vision of your future that integrates this transition experience while preserving core identity elements

This integrated approach fosters psychological stability during the transition, enabling you to maintain your core sense of self while developing effective management strategies for biological changes.

The cognitive dissonance between chronological identity and biological experience creates real challenges, but with strategic management, it need not destroy your established self-concept. By distinguishing between biological processes and core identity, avoiding common mistakes in identity preservation, and actively protecting your most essential self-concept elements, you can navigate this unexpected transition while maintaining psychological continuity.

In the next chapter, you'll discover how identifying your unique symptom patterns transforms perimenopause from a chaotic experience into a predictable and manageable one, creating the practical foundation for the identity preservation strategies outlined here.

CHAPTER 3. FINDING ORDER IN CHAOS

Your symptoms speak a language you haven't yet learned to understand.

For too many women experiencing early perimenopause, each day feels like walking through an unpredictable minefield of symptoms that strike without warning. This sense of randomness creates profound helplessness, as if your body has betrayed you with its apparent chaos. Yet beneath this seeming disorder lies a hidden structure—a pattern as unique to you as your fingerprint.

Dismantling the Myth of Random Perimenopause Symptoms

Sarah, a 38-year-old marketing executive, first noticed her symptoms at a critical client presentation. "I suddenly felt a wave of heat spread across my chest and up my neck. My heart started racing, and I completely lost my train of thought," she recalls. "The next week, the same thing happened during my daughter's school concert. I genuinely thought I was having panic attacks or some weird stress response—until it kept happening, seemingly at random."

This perception of randomness is one of the most damaging aspects of early perimenopause. When symptoms appear to strike without rhyme or reason, you lose your sense of control and ability to plan. Medical literature and popular media often reinforce this myth by describing perimenopause as an inherently chaotic time—a storm you must weather until it passes.

This portrayal isn't merely inaccurate—it's actively harmful. Research reveals that while perimenopause symptoms may seem random at first glance, they follow distinct patterns unique to each woman. These patterns originate from hormonal fluctuations that interact with your specific lifestyle factors, nutritional status, stress levels, and genetic makeup.

The myth of randomness persists for three main reasons:

1. Insufficient tracking: Most women don't document their symptoms thoroughly enough to identify patterns, viewing each occurrence as an isolated event rather than part of a sequence.

2. Medical oversight: Healthcare providers rarely help patients connect the dots between seemingly unrelated symptoms, missing opportunities to identify underlying hormonal patterns.

3. Pattern complexity: Your symptom patterns may be complex, with multiple influencing factors that make them challenging to detect without systematic tracking and analysis.

This shift from perceived chaos to identified patterns creates a foundation for everything else in your perimenopause management strategy. When you understand that your symptoms follow predictable patterns, you gain the power to predict, prepare for, and often prevent their most severe manifestations.

Identifying Your Symptom Patterns and Triggers

Melissa, a 41-year-old university professor, spent six months convinced her cognitive symptoms were early-onset dementia before discovering they followed a clear monthly pattern. "I noticed I consistently had word-finding difficulties and concentration problems during specific weeks of my cycle. Even though my periods were still regular, my brain wasn't functioning the same way throughout the month."

Your unique symptom patterns will reveal themselves when you implement a structured tracking system. This doesn't mean obsessively documenting every bodily sensation—it means strategically recording key data points that help you connect cause and effect.

The Essential Tracking Elements:

- Symptom specifics: What exactly did you experience? Be precise about the nature, location, and sensation.

- Timing details: What time of day? What day of your cycle (if applicable)? What day of the week?

- Intensity rating: How severe was the symptom on a scale of 1-10?

- Preceding factors: What did you eat, drink, or do in the 3-6 hours before?

- Environmental conditions: What was your stress level, sleep quality, and activity level?

- Alleviation factors: What helped reduce the symptom? What made it worse?

Dr. Serena Chen, reproductive endocrinologist, advises using both digital and analogue tracking methods: "Many of my patients combine a simple app for basic cycle tracking with a dedicated journal for more detailed symptom documentation. The physical act of writing often helps women notice connections they might miss when just tapping on a screen."

Pattern recognition becomes easier when you know what to look for. Common pattern types include:

1. Cycle-based patterns. Even with irregular periods, many early perimenopause symptoms follow predictable hormonal fluctuations. Track symptoms about your cycle, even if it's becoming less predictable. You may notice cognitive symptoms worsening during your luteal phase or sleep disruptions increasing around ovulation.

2. Time-of-day patterns. Hormonal fluctuations often follow daily rhythms. Some women experience worse hot flashes in the evening, while others notice mood changes that predictably strike mid-afternoon.

3. Trigger-response patterns. Certain foods, beverages, activities, or environmental factors consistently trigger or worsen specific symptoms. Common triggers include:

- Caffeine consumption (particularly afternoon intake)
- Alcohol (especially red wine and spirits)
- Sugar and refined carbohydrates
- Skipped meals leading to blood sugar drops
- Environmental temperature changes
- High-stress events or deadline pressure
- Disrupted sleep schedules
- Certain exercise timing or intensity

When Julia, a 39-year-old financial analyst, began tracking her triggers, she made a surprising discovery: "My worst brain fog consistently happened 30-45 minutes after my morning coffee, especially if I hadn't eaten protein with breakfast. Switching to a smaller coffee with a protein-rich breakfast completely changed my cognitive function."

This focus on pattern identification transforms your experience from helpless victim to informed investigator. By collecting your symptom data, you create a powerful resource for understanding your body's unique responses and developing targeted intervention strategies.

Projecting Your Symptom Trajectory Based on Patterns

Rachel, 43, had been tracking her early perimenopause symptoms for nine months when she noticed something significant: "I realised I could predict exactly when I'd experience sleep disruption based on my cycle. Even more importantly, I could see which symptoms were gradually increasing in intensity month by month, versus which ones remained stable."

This distinction between cyclical and progressive symptoms provides valuable insight into your perimenopause trajectory. While every woman's path through this transition is unique, pattern recognition allows you to create an informed projection of what lies ahead.

Cyclical symptoms recur in predictable patterns related to hormonal fluctuations within your menstrual cycle, even as that cycle becomes less regular. These symptoms might include:

- Mood changes that worsen premenstrual
- Sleep disturbances that peak during specific cycle phases
- Cognitive function changes that follow hormonal ebbs and flows
- Energy fluctuations tied to predictable hormonal shifts

Progressive symptoms gradually increase in frequency, intensity, or duration over time, exhibiting a trajectory rather than a cyclical pattern. Examples include:

- Gradual changes in menstrual regularity (cycles becoming shorter, then increasingly irregular)
- Persistent sleep disturbance

- Ongoing weight gain
- Decreased sexual interest
- Symptoms that do not resolve with the end of a menstrual cycle and tend to accumulate over time

By distinguishing between these two types, you can begin to chart your personal perimenopause progression. This projection isn't about predicting precisely what will happen—it's about recognising the patterns that emerge in your experience and preparing accordingly.

To create your symptom projection:

1. Review three months of tracking data to identify which symptoms follow cyclical patterns versus progressive trends.
2. Chart intensity changes for each symptom. Are specific symptoms steadily worsening while others remain stable?
3. Note frequency shifts. Are some symptoms occurring more often than when they first appeared?
4. Document duration changes. Are episodes of specific symptoms lasting longer than they initially did?
5. Connect to life events. How do your symptoms interact with predictable stress points in your calendar?

This analysis enables you to create a personalised projection that helps you prepare for what is likely ahead. Knowing that your cognitive function typically dips during certain hormonal phases allows you to schedule essential presentations or decisions outside those windows. Recognising that your sleep disruption is following a progressive pattern prompts you to prioritise sleep hygiene and supportive interventions.

The power of projection isn't in perfect prediction—it's in replacing fear of the unknown with informed preparation.

When you can anticipate likely symptom patterns, you transform from someone who's constantly surprised by your body to someone who works strategically with its patterns.

This shift from chaos to pattern recognition is the essential foundation for everything else in your perimenopause management approach. Understanding your unique symptom language enables you to transition from reactive suffering to a proactive approach.

In the next chapter, we'll build on this pattern recognition by exploring how to become your medical advocate, using your symptom data to secure appropriate care even when facing scepticism or dismissal. With your symptom patterns identified, you'll be equipped to communicate effectively with healthcare providers and advocate for the specific support you need.

CHAPTER 4.
BECOMING YOUR
OWN MEDICAL
ADVOCATE

Healthcare systems worldwide consistently
fail younger women with hormonal issues.

Women in their thirties and early forties experiencing perimenopause symptoms face a uniquely frustrating challenge within medical settings. Physicians trained to recognise these symptoms in women over fifty often dismiss identical symptoms in younger women as stress, anxiety, or depression. This systematic failure leaves thousands of women misdiagnosed, untreated, and questioning their perceptions. Medical gaslighting isn't just harmful—it blocks access to treatments that could restore your quality of life.

Why Conventional Medical Approaches
Fail Early Perimenopause Patients

Sarah, a 37-year-old marketing executive, visited five different doctors over eighteen months before receiving her perimenopause diagnosis. Each appointment followed a similar pattern: she described her symptoms—night sweats, brain fog, irregular periods, and mood swings—only to be told she was "too young" for perimenopause. Two doctors prescribed antidepressants without running hormone tests. Another suggested that she reduce her work hours to manage stress. The fourth recommended therapy is for "work-life balance issues."

The final doctor, a gynaecologist with specialised training in midlife women's health, ordered comprehensive hormone panels that confirmed what Sarah had suspected all along. Her Estrogen was fluctuating wildly, and her progesterone was low —classic perimenopause patterns regardless of age.

Sarah's experience exemplifies why conventional medical approaches consistently fail early perimenopause patients:

1. Age-based diagnostic bias creates a blind spot for symptoms occurring "too early"

2. Knowledge gaps in medical education mean many providers receive minimal training on perimenopause, with even less focus on early-onset cases

3. Symptom overlap with other conditions leads to misdiagnosis when age is used as the primary diagnostic filter

4. Reliance on outdated research that established menopause timing norms based on limited population studies from decades ago

5. Fragmented care models where symptoms affecting different body systems are treated separately without recognising the hormonal connection

This table highlights the stark contrast between how perimenopause symptoms are perceived in women of different ages:

Symptom	Interpretation in Women 50+	Interpretation in Women 35-45
Night	Likely hormonal,	Anxiety, overwork,

sweats	perimenopause	stress
Brain fog	Age-related cognitive changes, hormonal	Depression, sleep deprivation, and burnout
Mood swings	Hormonal fluctuations	Work stress, relationship issues, and the need for therapy
Irregular periods	Expected perimenopause change	Stress, thyroid issues, and diet
Sleep disruption	Hormonal changes	Poor sleep hygiene, anxiety, and too much screen time

The medical system isn't designed to help you, which means you must become your advocate. Let's explore how.

Medical Terminology That Commands Provider Respect and Attention

When Lisa first experienced brain fog and fatigue, she told her doctor she was "feeling fuzzy-headed and wiped out." The doctor nodded sympathetically but made no notes. At her next appointment, after researching medical terminology, Lisa instead reported "experiencing cognitive dysfunction including word-finding difficulties and short-term memory impairment, alongside persistent fatigue unrelieved by rest." The doctor's approach changed completely—he took detailed notes and ordered comprehensive testing.

The language you use fundamentally changes how medical providers perceive your symptoms. Vague descriptions trigger the "stressed woman" stereotype, while precise medical terminology signals that you're informed and should be taken seriously.

Essential terminology that commands clinical respect:

- Instead of "mood swings," say: "I'm experiencing mood lability with periods of heightened emotional reactivity followed by low mood states."

- Instead of "brain fog," say: "I'm experiencing cognitive dysfunction, including executive function deficits and working memory impairment that impacts my professional performance."

- Instead of "irregular periods," say: "My menstrual cycle has become irregular with variable cycle length ranging from 21 to 48 days and changes in flow volume and duration."

- Instead of "night sweats," say: "I'm experiencing nocturnal vasomotor symptoms that disrupt my sleep architecture, occurring approximately 3-4 times weekly."

- Instead of "tired all the time," say: "I'm experiencing persistent fatigue and reduced stamina unrelieved by adequate rest and nutrition."

This advanced terminology serves two crucial functions: it bypasses the dismissal filter many providers apply to younger women reporting perimenopause symptoms, and it demonstrates your informed status, making it harder for providers to offer simplified explanations or dismissals.

Keep a small reference card with these terms in your purse or phone notes to review before appointments. Practice saying these terms aloud so they come naturally during consultations. Remember, you're not trying to diagnose yourself—you're communicating symptoms in language that receives medical attention.

Identifying Knowledgeable Medical Providers

and Avoiding Dismissive Ones

After her third dismissed complaint about night sweats and mood changes, Jennifer developed a strategic approach to finding the right doctor. She researched specialists with additional training in perimenopause management, read patient reviews focusing on women under 45, and prepared specific questions to evaluate new providers' knowledge about early perimenopause. Within two appointments, she found a physician who not only validated her experience but offered a comprehensive treatment plan.

Not all healthcare providers are equal when it comes to recognising and treating early perimenopause. Selecting the right medical team requires thorough research and careful evaluation.

How to identify knowledgeable providers:

1. **Seek specific credentials and training**
   - Look for providers with additional certifications in women's midlife health
   - Search for membership in organisations like the North American Menopause Society (NAMS)
   - Check for physicians who list "perimenopause" (not just menopause) as a speciality area

2. **Research before booking**
   - Read patient reviews with attention to age-specific comments
   - Look for practices that mention early perimenopause on their websites
   - Check if they offer hormone testing as a standard service

3. **Conduct provider interviews**
   - Ask about their experience treating

perimenopause in women under 45

- Inquire about their typical approach to hormone testing
- Question their perspective on age requirements for perimenopause diagnosis

4. **Red flags that signal a potentially dismissive provider:**

- Uses phrases like "you're too young to worry about that"

- Suggests psychological causes before running physical tests

- Dismisses hormone testing as "unnecessary" based solely on age

- Recommends only lifestyle changes when symptoms are significantly impacting your life

- Shows impatience with detailed symptom descriptions

Remember, you're not just a patient—you're a consumer hiring a medical professional for their expertise. If you don't receive appropriate care, you have every right to seek another provider. Many women report needing to see 3-5 different physicians before finding one knowledgeable about early perimenopause.

Essential Lab Tests and How to Interpret Your Results

When Melissa finally convinced her doctor to run hormone tests, she received a brief message: "Your labs came back normal." Unsatisfied, she requested copies of her actual lab reports and discovered that her oestradiol levels were at the absolute bottom of the normal range. At the same time, her FSH was elevated—a classic perimenopause pattern her doctor had missed.

Standard "normal" lab ranges aren't designed to detect the hormonal fluctuations of perimenopause. Learning to interpret your results gives you critical information for self-advocacy.

Essential lab tests to request:

1. **Complete Hormone Panel**
   - Follicle Stimulating Hormone (FSH)
   - Oestradiol (E2)
   - Progesterone
   - Testosterone (Total and Free)
   - DHEA-S
   - Thyroid panel (TSH, Free T3, Free T4, TPO antibodies)
   - Cortisol (preferably through 4-point saliva testing)

2. **Supporting Tests**
   - Complete Blood Count (CBC)
   - Comprehensive Metabolic Panel (CMP)
   - Inflammatory markers (hsCRP, ESR)
   - Vitamin D levels
   - Vitamin B12 and folate
   - Iron studies, including ferritin

How to interpret your results:

Standard reference ranges on lab tests represent the middle 95% of the population tested, not optimal levels, and certainly not what is normal for your body. When reviewing your results:

- **Ask for actual numbers**, not just "normal" or "abnormal" assessments

- **Compare your current results to your baseline** if you have previous labs

- **Look for values at the extreme ends of "normal" ranges**
- **Track patterns over time** rather than focusing on single measurements
- **Pay attention to ratios** between hormones (particularly Estrogen to progesterone)

For FSH specifically, values between 10-25 IU/L can indicate early perimenopause even when your doctor might call them "normal." Oestradiol levels that fluctuate significantly between tests can be more telling than consistently low readings.

Key insight: Perimenopause is characterised by fluctuation, not absolute values. Single tests often fail to capture the pattern, which is why tracking over time is crucial.

Documentation Strategies That Transform Dismissal into Diagnosis

After months of having her symptoms dismissed, Rebecca developed a strategic approach to her medical appointments. She created a detailed symptom journal with specific metrics, charts showing symptom patterns, and a concise medical summary document. At her next appointment, she presented these materials with confidence. Her new gynaecologist spent twenty minutes reviewing her documentation and remarked, "This is incredibly helpful—I can see exactly what's happening." Rebecca received appropriate testing and treatment that same day.

Adequate documentation transforms vague complaints into compelling evidence that's difficult to dismiss.

Documentation tools that command medical attention:

1. **Symptom Journal**
   - Track frequency, intensity, duration, and triggers
   - Use numeric scales (1-10) to quantify

severity

- Note correlations with your cycle and other patterns
- Include impact on daily functioning and quality of life

2. **Cycle Tracking Apps and Charts**
   - Document menstrual cycle length, flow volume, and symptoms
   - Print out 6-12 months of data to show patterns
   - Highlight cycle irregularities and symptom clusters

3. **Medical Encounter Preparation Form**
   - Create a one-page summary of your top concerns
   - List symptoms in order of impact on your life
   - Include specific questions you need answered
   - Request specific tests you want considered

4. **Medical History Portfolio**
   - Compile previous relevant test results
   - Include family history focusing on hormonal health
   - List current medications and supplements
   - Note failed treatments or approaches already tried

The most effective documentation is concise, organised, and quantitative. Doctors respond to numbers, patterns, and clarity. Your goal is to present information in a format that mirrors medical thinking—systematic, evidence-based, and focused on measurable data.

How to present your documentation effectively:

- Begin appointments by saying, "I've prepared some information to help us use our time efficiently."

- Provide a concise overview before sharing detailed documentation.

- Use phrases like "I've tracked these symptoms for X months" to establish the thoroughness of your approach.

- When presenting symptom patterns, connect them explicitly to possible hormonal fluctuations.

- Ask directly: "Based on this documentation, what tests would you recommend evaluating for perimenopause?"

Remember, your documentation creates a medical record that becomes part of your official chart. This record creates accountability and can help overcome the initial dismissal many women face.

The Transformation from Dismissed Patient to Healthcare Partner

Your goal isn't just to receive a proper diagnosis and treatment —it's to establish yourself as an equal partner in your healthcare decisions. This transformation requires confidence, preparation, and persistence.

Steps to establish yourself as a healthcare partner:

1. **Speak the language of medicine**
   - Use precise terminology
   - Reference relevant research
   - Frame questions in terms of scientific evidence

2. **Bring solutions, not just problems**
   - Research treatment options before

appointments

- Ask specific questions about particular approaches
- Propose a collaborative plan rather than waiting for directives

3. **Set clear expectations**
    - Begin appointments by stating your goals
    - Clarify what you need from each encounter
    - Follow up consistently on agreed actions

4. **Build your medical team strategically**
    - Different providers for different needs
    - Coordinate your care across specialities
    - Inform providers about each other's recommendations

The transformation from dismissed patient to healthcare partner shifts the entire dynamic of your medical care. When providers recognise your informed status, they're more likely to engage with you as a collaborator rather than a passive recipient of care.

As we move into the next chapter on "The Protocol Paradigm Shift," you'll learn how to take this new healthcare partnership beyond simple advocacy into a systematic approach for managing your perimenopause experience. The medical system's limitations make self-directed protocols essential, and your ability to work effectively with healthcare providers forms the foundation for implementing these protocols successfully.

CHAPTER 5.
THE PROTOCOL
PARADIGM SHIFT

*Your body's unexpected rebellion demands
a considered response, not resignation.*

Most women experiencing early perimenopause find themselves caught in a cycle of dismissal, receiving generic advice that fails to address their unique challenges. This dismissal often comes from medical professionals, friends, family, and even their internal voices telling them to endure what's happening simply. The path forward isn't through passive acceptance, but through structured and systematic action.

Why Passive Approaches to
Perimenopause Management Fail

Rebecca, a 38-year-old marketing director, spent eighteen months following conventional advice about her symptoms: "get more sleep," "reduce stress," and "eat healthier." Despite these efforts, her brain fog worsened, hot flashes became more frequent, and her confidence in managing client presentations deteriorated.

"I was doing everything right," she explained during our consultation. "Yoga three times weekly, eight hours of sleep, Mediterranean diet, limited alcohol—all the standard wellness boxes checked. Yet my symptoms kept getting worse, and my doctor just suggested I meditate more."

Rebecca's experience highlights a fundamental truth: passive approaches to early perimenopause fail for three critical reasons:

1. **Timing mismatch**: Generic advice assumes you have decades to adjust, but early transitioners face immediate professional and personal demands requiring rapid symptom management.

2. **Intensity disconnect**: Standard recommendations aren't calibrated for the severity of symptoms that occur in a body unprepared for hormonal fluctuations, which can happen a decade earlier than expected.

3. **Context blindness**: Conventional guidance overlooks the unique life stage of early transitioners, who face peak career challenges simultaneously with hormonal disruptions.

This pattern repeats across my client practice, with women making dedicated efforts toward wellness approaches while watching their symptoms progress unchecked. The missing element? A structured protocol approach that matches the intensity and urgency of early perimenopause.

The Critical Difference Between General Wellness Advice and Targeted Protocols

General wellness advice and targeted protocols differ fundamentally in their approach, precision, and outcomes. This distinction is particularly significant for women navigating early perimenopause.

Aspect	General Wellness Advice	Targeted Protocols

Approach	Broad recommendations for overall health	Specific actions addressing individual symptom patterns
Timing	Ongoing, indefinite lifestyle adjustments	Intentional interventions linked to hormonal cycling
Precision	Generic one-size-fits-all suggestions	Customised to individual symptom clusters
Measurement	Vague markers of success	Clear metrics for tracking effectiveness
Focus	Whole-body wellness	Priority on identity-threatening symptoms
Action triggers	Calendar-based (daily/weekly)	Symptom pattern-based (reactive and proactive)
Evidence base	Generalised health research	Specific hormonal transition research
Professional input	Minimal, usually self-directed	Expert guidance and customisation

Consider Sarah, a 42-year-old financial analyst experiencing debilitating brain fog during client meetings. The general wellness advice she received—"get more sleep"—failed to address the timing of her cognitive symptoms, which followed a clear pattern related to her hormonal cycling.

Once Sarah implemented a targeted protocol with specific nutritional interventions timed to her cycle, cognitive enhancement techniques before key meetings, and planned scheduling of high-stakes work around her pattern, her professional performance stabilised.

The difference wasn't that Sarah wasn't "trying hard enough" with wellness approaches. The difference was that wellness approaches weren't designed for the specific challenge of hormone-driven cognitive symptoms threatening professional competence.

Contrasting Early vs. Conventional Perimenopause Management Needs

Early perimenopause creates fundamentally different management requirements compared to conventional (later-life) perimenopause. Understanding these distinctions helps explain why approaches effective for women in their 50s often fail for those experiencing transition a decade earlier.

Life Stage Differences

Women experiencing perimenopause at the expected time (late 40s to 50s) typically have:

- Established career positions with more flexibility and authority
- Children who are older or independent
- Greater financial security and professional stability
- Peer groups experiencing similar transitions

- A life narrative that aligns with biological changes

In contrast, early transitioners face:

- Peak career advancement stages require maximum cognitive performance
- Active parenting of young children or recent family formation
- Critical income-earning years for long-term financial planning
- Isolation from peers who cannot relate to their experience
- Profound cognitive dissonance between life stage and biological status

These contextual differences create entirely different management priorities. While women in conventional perimenopause may focus primarily on symptom relief, early transitioners must simultaneously preserve professional trajectory, maintain family stability, and protect core identity.

Jennifer, 37, described her experience: "When my mother went through this in her 50s, she could take mental health days when needed. She was established in her career. But I'm up for partnership next year—I can't afford a single day of appearing anything less than 100% competent."

Management Approach Differences

Conventional perimenopause management typically emphasises:

- Gradual lifestyle modifications
- Acceptance-based approaches to life changes
- Lower-intensity interventions with longer implementation timelines
- Focus on physical symptom management (hot

flashes, sleep disturbances)

- Less urgency around cognitive symptom treatment

Early perimenopause requires:

- Rapid implementation of effective protocols
- Identity preservation approaches alongside symptom management
- Higher intensity, more precisely targeted interventions
- Prioritisation of cognitive symptom management
- Planned career protection measures

This fundamental mismatch explains why generic perimenopause advice fails women experiencing it early—the approaches weren't designed for your specific context, timeline, or priorities.

Why Your Professional Position Requires Preservation, Not Just Symptom Relief

The stakes of cognitive symptoms are substantially higher during early perimenopause. This isn't just about comfort—it's about safeguarding your career trajectory during its most critical phase.

Most women experience peak earning potential and career advancement opportunities between the ages of 35 and 45, precisely when early perimenopause can strike. Cognitive symptoms during this phase don't merely create discomfort; they threaten:

- **Performance during evaluations**: Promotion and advancement often depend on demonstrating peak cognitive function during high-stakes presentations, projects, and reviews.
- **Leadership perception**: Executive presence requires

consistent mental sharpness, emotional regulation, and confident decision-making—all affected by hormonal fluctuations.

- **Long-term earning trajectory**: Studies show that career interruptions or performance declines during mid-career years create earnings gaps that rarely close in subsequent decades.

- **Opportunity access**: Being passed over for key projects or roles due to temporary cognitive symptoms can have a lasting impact on career paths.

Unlike women experiencing perimenopause at conventional ages who may have established their professional position, early transitioners face these symptoms precisely when career momentum is most critical.

Alexa, a 39-year-old tech executive, shared: "I built my reputation on quick thinking and innovative problem-solving. Suddenly, I was stuttering in presentations and forgetting key points. It wasn't just embarrassing—it threatened everything I'd worked for."

This reality demands an approach that goes beyond managing symptoms to preserving professional function. General wellness advice typically addresses how you feel; targeted protocols, on the other hand, address what you can do and who you continue to be despite biological changes.

Introduction to the BICEP Framework as Your Structured Solution

The BICEP Framework represents a structured solution designed explicitly for early perimenopause management, addressing both biological symptom control and chronological identity preservation simultaneously.

The framework arose from years of working with hundreds of women experiencing early transition, identifying consistent patterns in what worked versus what failed. The approach differs fundamentally from conventional perimenopause management by focusing equally on symptom management and identity preservation.

BICEP stands for:

Baseline: Establishing your starting point and pattern recognition system. **I**ntervention: Implementing targeted protocols matched to your specific symptoms. **C**ommunication: Developing effective plans for critical relationships. **E**valuation: Measuring progress and refining your approach. **P**rojection: Creating your integrated future self

This framework transforms early perimenopause management from a scattershot collection of wellness tips to a planned, systematic approach addressing your specific challenges.

Each element of the framework works together to create a continuous feedback loop, enabling adaptation as your symptoms change and your needs evolve. Unlike passive approaches that leave you reacting to symptoms as they arise, the BICEP Framework puts you in a proactive position.

Women who implement this structured protocol approach report three key outcomes:

1. **Symptom predictability**: Rather than being ambushed by symptoms, they develop the ability to anticipate and prepare for fluctuations in their symptoms.

2. **Identity continuity**: They maintain their core sense of self despite biological changes, preserving professional effectiveness and relationship quality.

3. **Progressive mastery**: They develop increasing confidence in their ability to navigate this transition effectively, transforming from victim to navigator.

Rachel, 41, described her experience after implementing the

framework: "For the first time in two years, I feel like myself again—not because my symptoms disappeared, but because I have systems to manage them effectively. I'm no longer at the mercy of my hormones; I have plans that work."

The fundamental promise of the BICEP Framework is transformation from helplessness to effectiveness—from being controlled by unpredictable symptoms to purposefully managing your transition.

From Victim to Navigator: The Protocol-Based Mindset Shift

At the heart of effective early perimenopause management lies a critical mindset shift. This transition isn't about surrendering to biological change but developing systematic approaches to navigate it while preserving what matters most.

The passive approach positions you as a victim—someone to whom perimenopause happens, who must simply endure its effects until they eventually pass. The protocol-based approach positions you as a navigator—someone who acknowledges the biological reality while implementing deliberate systems to maintain control of your trajectory.

This shift requires:

- **Accepting reality while rejecting helplessness**: Acknowledging that your hormones are changing while dismissing the notion that you must passively accept all consequences

- **Prioritising evidence over anecdote**: Moving beyond well-meaning but ineffective generic advice to approaches backed by research and targeted to your specific needs

- **Embracing pattern recognition**: Shifting from seeing symptoms as random chaos to recognising them as following predictable patterns unique to your body

- **Adopting calculated timing**: Learning to align interventions, work demands, and energy expenditure with your hormonal patterns rather than fighting against them

- **Moving from secrecy to selective disclosure**: Developing clear tactics for when, how, and with whom to discuss your transition to secure needed support

This mindset shift forms the foundation for all protocol implementations. Without it, even the most effective policies become merely mechanical techniques rather than components of a coherent management approach.

In the next chapter, we'll explore the philosophical foundation of the BICEP Framework—how it specifically addresses the unique challenge of integrating unexpected biological changes with your chronological identity and life stage.

We'll examine how this structured approach transforms early perimenopause from an identity-threatening disruption to a manageable transition that can be navigated well. You'll discover how the framework provides not just symptom relief, but a comprehensive way to maintain your core sense of self while adapting to changing biological realities.

CHAPTER 6. THE BIOLOGICAL- CHRONOLOGICAL INTEGRATION FRAMEWORK

Integration begins where acceptance
ends, and agency takes hold.

When your body sends signals that contradict your chronological identity, the natural response is resistance. You push back against these changes, hoping they'll disappear or at least delay their intrusion into your life. This resistance, while understandable, consumes precious energy and deepens the disconnect between your chronological self-concept and biological reality. The path forward requires neither surrender nor battle, but strategic integration.

The Philosophy of Integration Over Acceptance

Most conventional wisdom about perimenopause centres on acceptance, encouraging women to "embrace the change" or "surrender to the transition." This passive approach fails spectacularly for early transitioners like you.

Acceptance implies giving up—relinquishing your established identity and submitting to a biological process you didn't choose and certainly didn't expect so soon. That's why women in their 30s and early 40s often react with such intense resistance to perimenopause symptoms. Your rejection isn't mere denial; it's a valid protection of your chronological identity.

Integration, by contrast, honours both realities simultaneously:

- Your chronological identity as a vital woman in her prime years
- Your biological experience of hormonal transition

Rather than forcing you to choose between these competing truths, integration creates a framework that allows both to coexist. This philosophy underpins every aspect of the approach you're about to learn.

Integration means maintaining your core identity while developing strategic responses to biological changes that occur over time. It allows you to say: "Yes, my body is experiencing hormonal fluctuations typically associated with older women, AND I remain the same capable professional, engaged parent, and vibrant individual I've always been."

This AND stance, rather than the EITHER/OR approach most women are offered, creates the psychological space needed to navigate early perimenopause without identity crisis.

The BICEP Framework: Your Structured Path Forward

The Biological-Chronological Integration Framework—or BICEP Framework—provides the structured approach you've been searching for. It transforms overwhelming chaos into manageable steps while preserving your core identity.

The framework consists of five sequential steps:

1. **Baseline**: Establishing your symptom patterns and

    identity foundations

2. **I**ntervention: Implementing targeted protocols for your unique symptom clusters

3. **C**ommunication: Developing strategic approaches for critical relationships

4. **E**valuation: Measuring progress and refining your approach

5. **P**rojection: Creating your integrated future self

Each step builds on the previous one, creating a continuous cycle of assessment, action, and refinement. This isn't a one-time process but an ongoing system you'll use throughout your transition.

The acronym "BICEP" isn't accidental—it represents strength in the face of challenge. Just as a physical bicep muscle allows you to lift and carry weight, this framework gives you the strength to carry the weight of early transition without buckling under its pressure.

How Structured Protocols Transform Chaos

Perhaps the most disorienting aspect of early perimenopause is its unpredictability. Symptoms seem to appear randomly, without a pattern or warning, leaving you perpetually off balance.

This perceived randomness creates psychological distress beyond the physical symptoms themselves. Humans are pattern-seeking creatures—we can endure significant challenges when we understand their parameters and can predict their occurrence. It's the unpredictability, more than the symptoms themselves, that creates the sense of helplessness many early transitioners describe.

Structured protocols eliminate this randomness by creating recognisable patterns and standardised responses. They transform your experience from chaotic crisis to predictable process in three key ways:

1. Pattern Recognition

The Baseline step teaches you to identify your unique symptom patterns, helping you see the underlying order in what feels like chaos. You'll learn to recognise trigger factors, cyclical patterns, and symptom clusters specific to your body.

2. Strategic Response

With patterns identified, the Intervention step provides targeted protocols matched to your specific symptoms. This eliminates the exhausting trial-and-error approach most women take, replacing it with evidence-based strategies.

3. Progress Tracking

The Evaluation step creates objective metrics to measure your progress, transforming subjective feelings into measurable data. This allows you to refine your approach based on evidence rather than emotion.

Together, these elements create a structure that counters the fundamental chaos of early perimenopause. Rather than being blindsided by symptoms, you'll develop the ability to anticipate and manage them proactively.

Setting Realistic Expectations

Before diving into the framework details, let's establish clear expectations about what this approach can and cannot do for you.

The BICEP Framework will:

- Help you identify and predict your unique symptom patterns
- Provide targeted strategies for managing specific symptoms
- Guide you in preserving your core identity through

transition

- Equip you with language and strategies for critical relationships
- Create a structured approach to an otherwise chaotic experience

The BICEP Framework will not:

- eliminate all perimenopause symptoms
- Work instantly without consistent implementation
- Replace with proper medical care when needed
- Offer a one-size-fits-all solution to symptoms

Implementation of this framework requires commitment. You'll need to dedicate time to tracking symptoms, applying interventions, and evaluating results. The payoff—maintaining your identity and managing symptoms while continuing your professional trajectory—makes this investment worthwhile, but it is an investment, nonetheless.

Most women see noticeable improvements within 30-45 days of consistent implementation, with significant transformation occurring around the 90-day mark. I recommend committing to the whole framework for at least three months before evaluating its effectiveness for your unique situation.

The Implementation Timeline

To help you plan your implementation journey, here's a realistic timeline for working through the BICEP Framework:

Phase	Timeframe	Focus	Expected Outcomes
Foundation	Weeks 1-2	Completing baseline assessments and establishing tracking systems	A clear understanding of your symptom patterns and identity priorities
Initial Implementation	Weeks 3-6	Beginning targeted interventions and communication strategies	First signs of symptom pattern predictability and initial symptom relief

| Refinement | Weeks 7-12 | Evaluating effectiveness and refining the approach | Significant symptom management improvement and growing confidence |
| Mastery | Month 4+ | Ongoing cycle of implementation with increasing sophistication | Integrated identity with managed symptoms and restored sense of control |

This timeline assumes consistent application of the framework principles. Progress isn't always linear—you may experience symptom flares or setbacks—but the overall trajectory should show improvement in both symptom management and identity integration.

Preparing for the Identity Preservation Journey

Identity preservation forms the core of this framework. While symptom management is essential, maintaining your sense of self through transition remains the primary goal.

To prepare for this journey, take a moment to reflect on these questions:

1. Which aspects of your identity feel most threatened by perimenopause symptoms?
2. What roles or capabilities define your core sense of self?
3. How has your relationship with your body changed since symptoms began?
4. What would successful navigation of this transition look like for you?

Your answers will guide your implementation of the framework, helping you prioritise interventions that protect your most essential identity elements.

Remember that identity preservation doesn't mean rigid attachment to every aspect of your pre-perimenopause self. Some flexibility allows for growth through this transition. The goal is to maintain continuity of your core self while accommodating biological changes.

Introducing the Five Framework Steps

Let's briefly examine each component of the BICEP Framework before exploring them in depth in subsequent chapters.

Baseline

This foundational step establishes your starting point across multiple dimensions:

- Symptom patterns, frequencies, and intensities
- Identity elements you consider essential to preserve
- Current energy levels, cognitive function, and emotional patterns
- Life priorities and responsibilities

Without this baseline, it is impossible to measure progress or identify effective interventions accurately. Many women skip this critical step in their haste for relief, only to find themselves unable to determine what's working and what isn't.

Intervention

With the baseline established, you'll implement targeted protocols for your specific symptom clusters:

- The Cognitive Preservation Protocol for brain fog and memory issues
- The Energy Allocation System for managing fluctuating energy
- The Hormonal Pattern Management system for anticipating symptoms

These aren't generic wellness tips, but instead structured approaches specifically designed for early perimenopause symptoms, with a particular emphasis on preserving professional function.

Communication

This often-overlooked step addresses how you'll discuss your experience with critical people in your life:

- Healthcare providers who may dismiss symptoms due to your age
- Partners who don't understand the changes you're experiencing
- Colleagues and supervisors who might misinterpret cognitive symptoms
- Children who notice changes but lack the framework to understand them

Strategic communication helps prevent unnecessary strain on relationships during an already challenging transition.

Evaluation

Regular assessment keeps your approach on track:

- Measuring intervention effectiveness with objective metrics
- Conducting Identity Continuity Reviews to ensure core self-preservation
- Refining protocols based on documented results
- Adjusting timelines and expectations as needed

This systematic evaluation transforms subjective experiences into actionable data, allowing for evidence-based refinement.

Projection

The final step creates a forward-focused vision:

- Developing your integrated future self-concept
- Creating a realistic transition timeline
- Identifying emerging strengths and capacities
- Reframing your transition narrative from disruption

to integration

This forward focus prevents you from becoming stuck in grief or resistance, helping you see perimenopause as a chapter in your story rather than an unwelcome interruption.

The Role of Identity Anchors

Throughout the implementation of the BICEP Framework, you'll use Identity Anchors—specific elements of your self-concept that remain stable despite physical changes. These anchors provide continuity during transition, reminding you of who you fundamentally are beyond hormonal fluctuations.

Standard Identity Anchors include:

- Core values and principles that guide your decisions
- Expertise and knowledge you've developed over the years
- Relationships that define essential aspects of your life
- Creative expressions that reflect your unique perspective
- Life accomplishments that biological changes can't erase

In the next chapter, you'll identify your personal Identity Anchors as part of establishing your baseline.

The BICEP Cycle

While the framework steps follow a sequential order, they also form a continuous cycle. After completing your first round of all five steps, you'll return to Baseline with new information, refine your Interventions based on Evaluation results, adjust your communication strategies as needed, and continue updating your Projection of your integrated self.

This cyclical approach allows for continuous refinement as

your symptoms evolve, and your mastery deepens. Early perimenopause isn't static—it changes over time, necessitating an adaptive strategy that develops in response to your experiences.

The BICEP Framework provides precisely this kind of flexible structure—rigid enough to create order from chaos, yet adaptable enough to accommodate your unique symptom pattern and identity needs.

Moving From Theory to Practice

Understanding the framework's philosophy and structure is just the beginning. The actual transformation comes through the consistent implementation of each step.

In the next chapter, we'll dive into the practical details of establishing your Baseline—the essential foundation for all subsequent work. You'll complete your Symptom Pattern Recognition Assessment, create your Identity Anchor Inventory, and establish the tracking systems that will reveal the patterns currently hidden in your experience.

This baseline work might seem less immediately rewarding than jumping straight to interventions, but it's the crucial groundwork that makes those interventions effective. By accurately mapping your unique symptom landscape and identity priorities now, you'll save countless hours of frustration and enable precisely targeted strategies moving forward.

CHAPTER 7.
BASELINE: CREATING
YOUR FOUNDATION

Knowledge begins with honest self-assessment and careful observation.

When you face the chaos of early perimenopause, the path forward isn't through immediate action or quick fixes. It starts with establishing clear reference points that anchor you through the transition. This foundation-setting step is what separates women who merely endure perimenopause from those who strategically navigate it. Your baseline becomes the compass that guides all future decisions.

Understanding Your Unique Symptom Patterns

"I never realised my symptoms followed a pattern until I started tracking them," explains Melissa, a 39-year-old marketing executive who began experiencing unexplained fatigue, brain fog, and night sweats at 37. "I thought everything was completely random. I'd have good days and bad days with no rhyme or reason."

Many women share Melissa's initial assumption. The seemingly unpredictable nature of early perimenopause symptoms creates a sense of helplessness that compounds the physical discomfort. Yet beneath this apparent chaos, patterns exist that can transform how you manage this transition.

The Symptom Pattern Recognition Assessment isn't simply about listing what you feel—it's about uncovering the hidden relationships between your symptoms, triggers, and timing. When you document these connections systematically, you gain control over what previously felt uncontrollable.

To begin your assessment, track these five core elements daily for at least 21 days:

1. **Symptom type and intensity** (rate each on a 1-10 scale)

2. **Time of day** symptoms appear or worsen

3. **Food intake** in the 3 hours before symptom onset

4. **Stress levels** (1-10 scale) throughout the day

5. **Sleep quality** from the previous night

This initial tracking period reveals your unique symptom clusters—combinations of symptoms that typically occur together. For instance, you might notice that brain fog, fatigue, and irritability often coincide, while hot flashes and night sweats form a separate cluster.

Symptom Cluster	Common Patterns	Tracking Focus
Cognitive symptoms (brain fog, memory issues, word-finding difficulties)	Often worse in the morning or after carbohydrate-heavy meals	Track meal timing/content and cognitive demands
Vasomotor symptoms (hot flashes, night sweats)	Frequently triggered by alcohol, spicy foods, or stress	Document food/drink consumption and stress

		levels
Mood fluctuations (irritability, anxiety, sadness)	May correlate with poor sleep or before vasomotor symptoms	Monitor sleep quality and symptom sequences
Energy fluctuations (fatigue, insomnia, afternoon crashes)	Often follow predictable daily patterns	Note energy levels throughout the day and sleep patterns

Jenna, a 41-year-old attorney, discovered through her symptom tracking that her brain fog wasn't random but followed a specific pattern: "It was always worst on Thursday mornings after my Wednesday evening wine with dinner, and before important meetings when my stress was high. Once I identified this pattern, I could plan around it—scheduling critical thinking tasks for Tuesdays and avoiding alcohol on nights before important workdays."

The assessment also helps distinguish between cyclical and progressive symptoms:

- **Cyclical symptoms** recur in patterns (daily, weekly, or monthly) and respond well to timing-based management strategies
- **Progressive symptoms** gradually increase in frequency or intensity over time and require escalating intervention approaches

Understanding this distinction is crucial—it determines whether you should focus on timing your activities around predictable symptom windows or implementing progressive intervention strategies.

Creating Your Identity Anchor Inventory

Early perimenopause often creates a sense of disconnection from your familiar self. The Identity Anchor Inventory serves as a conscious effort to preserve what matters most about who you are.

"I didn't Realise how much of my identity was tied to my mental sharpness until brain fog began affecting my work," shares Rachel, a 38-year-old financial analyst. "Creating my Identity Anchor Inventory helped me separate my essential self from these temporary symptoms."

Begin by documenting:

1. **Core values** that define you regardless of biological changes
2. **Essential roles** you wish to maintain through transition
3. **Self-concept elements** are most important to preserve
4. **Skills and strengths** you rely on regularly
5. **Personality traits** central to how you see yourself

This inventory isn't just a list—it's a declaration of what remains constant despite biological change. By explicitly naming these elements, you create psychological anchors that prevent identity erosion during episodes of symptoms.

Rebecca, a 42-year-old professor, found unexpected relief through this process: "Writing down that my analytical thinking, my role as a mentor, and my love of learning were core to who I am, regardless of hormonal fluctuations, gave me a sense of continuity I was missing. I could separate the fog in my brain from who I fundamentally am."

Your inventory should distinguish between identity elements that:

Category	Description	Examples
Permanent	Core aspects unlikely to change	Values, life philosophy, key relationships
Adaptable	Elements that can evolve while maintaining their essence	Work approaches, communication styles
Temporary	Aspects tied to specific life stages	Particular job positions, some physical capabilities

This categorisation helps you focus your preservation efforts where they matter most—on the permanent elements that define your core self.

Establishing Objective Baseline Measurements

Perimenopause symptoms can feel frustratingly subjective. Establishing quantifiable baselines transforms vague perceptions into trackable data points.

"My doctor kept dismissing my complaints because I couldn't precisely describe how my energy had changed," explains Alicia, a 40-year-old project manager. "Once I had baseline measurements and could say 'My ability to focus on complex tasks has decreased from 90 minutes to 45 minutes,' the conversation completely shifted."

For accurate baselining, measure:

1. **Cognitive function**
   - Reading comprehension time for standard material
   - Word recall capacity in 60 seconds
   - Time to complete familiar complex tasks
   - Working memory span

2. **Energy patterns**
   - Morning energy rating (1-10 scale)
   - Afternoon energy rating
   - Evening energy rating
   - Energy recovery time after exertion

3. **Emotional patterns**
   - Daily mood ratings (morning, afternoon, evening)
   - Emotional reactivity triggers
   - Recovery time after emotional events
   - Anxiety frequency and context

These measurements provide objective reference points that help you:

- Identify subtle changes before they become disruptive
- Document improvements from interventions
- Communicate effectively with healthcare providers
- Distinguish between normal fluctuations and significant shifts

Christine, a 36-year-old engineer, notes: "Having these measurements helped me stop questioning myself. When my ability to concentrate dropped from 50 minutes to 25 minutes, I could prove something real was happening—to my doctor and myself."

Creating Sustainable Tracking Systems

The key to effective tracking lies in striking a balance between comprehensive data and practical implementation. Many women abandon tracking because their systems are too complex or time-consuming.

"I tried tracking everything at first and gave up after three days," admits Laura, a 39-year-old retail manager. "The simpler system we developed—just three minutes morning and night—has given me insights I never expected."

Design your tracking system with these principles:

1. **Minimal time commitment** - Aim for under 5 minutes daily

2. **Integration with existing routines** - Attach tracking to habits you already have

3. **Focus on high-yield data** - Track what directly influences your decisions

4. **Visual organisation** - Use colour coding or symbols for quick pattern recognition

5. **Flexible format** - Choose digital or paper based on your preferences

For busy professionals, these streamlined approaches work best:

- **The 3-2-1 Method**: Track 3 symptoms, two triggers, and one intervention daily

- **Traffic Light System**: Rate key areas as green (good), yellow (caution), or red (problem) each morning and evening

- **Voice Memo Tracking**: Record brief observations that get transcribed weekly

- **Partner Observation**: Ask partners to note changes they observe in specific areas

These systems strike a balance between thoroughness and sustainability, ensuring you gather crucial data without adding stress to your already busy schedule.

Distinguishing Perimenopause from Other Conditions

Not every symptom you experience during this time is necessarily hormonal. Establishing a baseline helps determine whether symptoms stem from perimenopause or other health conditions.

"I assumed my heart palpitations were stress or perimenopause," shares Diane, a 41-year-old accountant. "My tracking showed they only happened after caffeine and had nothing to do with my hormonal patterns. It was such a relief to address the actual cause."

The Symptom Source Assessment Framework helps categorise symptoms by likely cause:

Characteristic	Likely Perimenopause	Possible Other Cause
Pattern	Fluctuates with hormonal cycles	Consistent regardless of the cycle
Triggers	Responds to hormone-influencing factors	Triggered by non-hormonal factors
Response	Improves with hormone-balancing approaches	Doesn't respond to hormonal strategies
Timing	Often follows sequential symptom patterns	Appears isolated from other symptoms
History	It may have appeared with other hormone shifts	No connection to past hormonal events

This framework doesn't replace medical diagnosis but provides clarity on which symptoms warrant specific medical attention versus hormonal management strategies.

Karen, a 38-year-old sales director, experienced this distinction firsthand: "I tracked my symptoms for a month and realised my joint pain followed a completely different pattern than my hot flashes and mood swings. I took this information to my doctor, who diagnosed an autoimmune condition completely separate from perimenopause. Now I'm getting proper treatment for both."

The baseline establishment process transforms your approach from reactive to strategic. By understanding your unique symptom patterns, anchoring your core identity, measuring objective changes, creating sustainable tracking systems, and distinguishing between hormonal and non-hormonal issues, you lay the foundation for all future management decisions.

This foundation doesn't just support symptom management —it preserves your sense of continuity through change. As you move forward with the targeted interventions in the next chapter, you'll build upon this baseline to implement protocols specifically matched to your unique symptom profile and personal priorities.

CHAPTER 8.
INTERVENTION:
TARGETED
PROTOCOLS FOR
YOUR SYMPTOM
PROFILE

---

*Your body speaks a language only
you can fully interpret.*

When symptoms arise, they communicate specific messages about your hormonal changes. These signals, once decoded through the baseline assessments you completed in the previous chapter, provide the foundation for targeted action. Understanding your unique patterns is only the first step; now it's time to respond with precision.

Shifting from Passive to Active Management

Most women experiencing early perimenopause find themselves caught in a cycle of reactive management. A hot flash strikes during an important meeting, and they frantically search for relief. Brain fog descends as they prepare for a presentation, sending them into a panic. Sleep disruption leaves them exhausted, reaching desperately for any solution promising rest.

This reactive approach is understandable but ultimately ineffective. Generic perimenopause advice rarely addresses the unique challenges of early transitioners, particularly those balancing demanding careers with family responsibilities. Women in their mid-30s to mid-40s cannot afford the trial-and-error approach that might be acceptable for those in their 50s, who have more flexibility and fewer professional demands.

The intervention stage of the BICEP Framework completely transforms this paradigm. Instead of reacting to symptoms as they arise, you'll implement strategic protocols calibrated to your specific symptom profile. This targeted approach dramatically increases effectiveness while minimising disruption to your daily life.

Prioritising Interventions Based on Identity Preservation Needs

Not all symptoms deserve equal attention. Some directly threaten your core identity and professional functioning, while others, though uncomfortable, may have less impact on what matters most to you. The key to effective intervention is prioritisation based on your unique identity preservation needs.

The Identity Impact Assessment

Begin by ranking your symptoms according to how significantly they threaten your most valued aspects of identity. Consider using this simple matrix:

Symptom	Identity Impact (1-10)	Professional Impact (1-10)	Relationship Impact (1-10)	Total Score
Brain fog				
Hot flashes				
Sleep disruptio				

n

Mood changes

Energy fluctuations

Memory issues

Complete this assessment by assigning scores to each symptom based on its significant impact on the three core areas. The highest total scores indicate where you should focus your intervention efforts first.

Case Study: Rebecca's Prioritisation

Rebecca, a 38-year-old marketing executive, completed her Identity Impact Assessment with these results:

Symptom	Identity Impact (1-10)	Professional Impact (1-10)	Relationship Impact (1-10)	Total Score
Brain fog	9	10	7	26
Hot flashes	6	8	4	18
Sleep disruption	8	9	7	24
Mood changes	7	6	9	22
Energy fluctuations	8	9	8	25
Memory	8	10	6	24

issues

Based on these scores, Rebecca prioritised interventions addressing brain fog, energy fluctuations, and sleep disruption —the three symptoms most threatening to her overall functioning and core identity.

Key Principle: Address Root Causes, Not Just Symptoms

When prioritising interventions, look for connections between symptoms that may indicate a common underlying cause. Often, addressing one root cause can improve multiple symptoms simultaneously. For example:

- Sleep disruption often contributes to brain fog and energy fluctuations

- Hormonal fluctuations may trigger both mood changes and hot flashes

- Nutritional deficiencies can exacerbate cognitive symptoms and energy levels

By identifying these connections, you can implement targeted protocols that address multiple symptoms with a single intervention strategy, maximising efficiency and results.

Implementing the Cognitive Preservation Protocol for Brain Fog and Memory Issues

For many professional women, cognitive symptoms represent the most alarming and disruptive aspect of early perimenopause. The sudden inability to recall information, focus on complex tasks, or articulate thoughts clearly can threaten professional competence and core identity.

The Cognitive Preservation Protocol provides a structured approach to maintaining mental clarity despite hormonal fluctuations. This protocol encompasses nutritional interventions, timing techniques, and compensatory systems that work in tandem to support cognitive function.

Nutritional Foundation for Cognitive Function

Research suggests that targeted nutritional approaches can significantly alleviate cognitive symptoms during perimenopause. The most effective strategy includes:

1. **Blood Sugar Stabilisation**: Irregular glucose levels exacerbate hormonal fluctuations that trigger brain fog. Implement these specific approaches:
   - Eat within 30 minutes of waking
   - Include protein with every meal and snack (minimum 15g)
   - Limit refined carbohydrates and sugar
   - Never go more than 4 hours without eating during waking hours

2. **Brain-Supporting Nutrients**: Certain nutrients specifically support neurotransmitter production and neural function:
   - Omega-3 fatty acids (aim for 1,000-2,000mg EPA/DHA daily)
   - B vitamins, particularly B6, B12, and folate
   - Magnesium (400-600mg daily, preferably as magnesium Threonate or glycinate)
   - Antioxidants from colourful vegetables and fruits

3. **Hormone-Balancing Foods**: Include foods that naturally support hormonal balance:
   - Phytoestrogens from ground flaxseed, organic soy, and legumes
   - Cruciferous vegetables (broccoli, cauliflower, Brussels sprouts)
   - Zinc-rich foods like oysters, pumpkin seeds, and grass-fed beef

Strategic Timing Techniques

Cognitive function typically follows predictable patterns throughout the day, with additional fluctuations based on your hormonal cycles. By mapping these patterns, you can strategically schedule activities requiring peak mental performance:

1. **Track Your Cognitive Peaks**: For 7-10 days, rate your mental clarity on a scale of 1-10 at these intervals:
   - Upon waking
   - Mid-morning (10-11 am)
   - Early afternoon (1-2 pm)
   - Late afternoon (4-5 pm)
   - Evening (7-8 pm)

2. **Map Against Hormonal Patterns**: Compare your cognitive tracking with your symptom journal to identify connections between hormonal fluctuations and cognitive function.

3. **Schedule Strategically**: Once you've identified your peak cognitive periods:
   - Schedule high-stakes professional activities during your consistent peak times
   - Reserve routine, less demanding tasks for lower cognitive function periods
   - Block your calendar to protect your peak performance times
   - Communicate these needs to colleagues when appropriate (we'll cover communication strategies in Chapter 9)

Compensatory Systems for Cognitive Protection

Even with optimal nutrition and strategic timing, cognitive symptoms will still occur during this transition. Implementing compensatory systems creates safety nets that protect your professional performance:

1. **External Memory Systems**: Reduce the cognitive load of remembering by implementing:
   - A centralised digital note system (using apps like Evernote, Notion, or OneNote)
   - Visual reminders and cues placed strategically in your environment
   - Recording capabilities for meetings and meaningful conversations (with appropriate permissions)
   - Standardised templates for recurring tasks and projects

2. **Cognitive Scaffolding Techniques**: These strategies support thinking processes during brain fog episodes:
   - Mind mapping for complex problems (use digital tools like MindMeister or XMind)
   - Decision matrices for important choices when executive function is compromised
   - Checklists for routine procedures that might be affected by memory lapses
   - Processing prompts: written questions that guide thinking when focus is difficult

3. **Emergency Protocols for Acute Cognitive Episodes**: Develop specific strategies for when brain fog strikes unexpectedly:
   - "Pause and breathe" technique: 4-7-8 breathing pattern for 60 seconds
   - Standardised language for requesting brief breaks during meetings
   - Quick reset activities (5-minute walk, cold water on wrists, peppermint tea)

○ Backup explanations for momentary lapses that maintain professional credibility

Case Study: Catherine's Cognitive Protocol Implementation

Catherine, a 42-year-old financial analyst, developed severe brain fog that threatened her ability to process complex numerical data—the core of her professional identity. After implementing the Cognitive Preservation Protocol, she made these key discoveries:

- Her cognitive function peaked consistently between 7-9 am, with a secondary peak from 4-6 pm
- Blood sugar drops dramatically worsened her brain fog
- Magnesium supplementation (500mg daily) significantly improved her word-finding ability
- Creating standardised analysis templates reduced cognitive load during symptom flares

Catherine restructured her schedule to perform complex analyses during her morning peak, implemented a protein-based breakfast and mid-morning snack protocol, added magnesium supplementation, and developed templates for recurring analyses. Within three weeks, her cognitive symptoms, while still present, no longer threatened her professional performance.

Developing Your Energy Allocation System for Strategic Resource Management

Next to cognitive symptoms, energy fluctuations represent the most significant challenge for early perimenopause management. The sudden onset of profound fatigue, unpredictable energy crashes, and reduced capacity often occurs while your life demands remain unchanged or even increase.

The Energy Allocation System provides a structured approach to managing limited energy reserves across competing demands. This system includes energy forecasting, strategic scheduling, and recovery techniques that maintain productivity while honouring your changing capacity.

Energy Mapping and Forecasting

Understanding your energy patterns allows you to predict and plan for fluctuations:

1. **Baseline Energy Assessment**: Using your symptom tracking data, identify:
   - Your average daily energy curve
   - Warning signs that precede energy crashes
   - Activities, foods, or environments that consistently drain or boost energy
   - Hormonal pattern connections to energy fluctuations

2. **Energy Budget Calculation**: Determine your current energy capacity:
   - Estimate your pre-perimenopause energy capacity as 100%
   - Assess your current capacity as a percentage of your previous baseline
   - Calculate separate budgets for physical, mental, and emotional energy

3. **Forecast Development**: Create weekly and monthly energy forecasts based on:
   - Hormonal cycle patterns identified in your baseline tracking
   - Known energy-intensive events on your calendar
   - Historical patterns from your symptom

journal

Strategic Energy Allocation

Once you understand your energy patterns, implement a system for strategic allocation:

1. **Priority-Based Allocation**: Distribute energy resources according to your core values:
    - Identify non-negotiable activities that align with your essential identity elements
    - Determine which activities can be modified, delegated, or eliminated
    - Create energy protection boundaries around your highest-priority commitments

2. **Capacity-Matched Scheduling**: Align your calendar with your energy forecast:
    - Schedule high-value, energy-intensive activities during predicted high-energy periods
    - Block recovery time following energy-intensive events
    - Build buffer zones around commitments during predicted low-energy phases
    - Implement a "minimum viable performance" approach for necessary activities during low-energy periods

3. **Strategic Rest Integration**: Rather than waiting until exhaustion forces rest, implement:
    - Scheduled micro-recovery periods (5-15 minutes) throughout each day
    - Specific restoration activities matched to your energy depletion pattern
    - Preventative rest is scheduled before anticipated energy-intensive events

- Clear boundaries between work and recovery periods

Energy Recovery and Renewal Techniques

Develop specific techniques for energy restoration appropriate for your symptom profile:

1. **Physical Energy Renewal**:
   - Movement snacks: 3-5 minute movement breaks every 60-90 minutes
   - Strategic hydration protocol (typically 75-100ml every 60-90 minutes)
   - Breath work techniques (box breathing, physiological sighing)
   - Power rest positions (modified legs-up-the-wall pose, supported recline)

2. **Mental Energy Renewal**:
   - Attention switching activities that use different neural pathways
   - Nature exposure (even brief viewing of natural scenes)
   - Sensory reset techniques (aromatherapy, temperature change, sound)
   - Cognitive load reduction strategies (noise-cancelling headphones, monotasking)

3. **Emotional Energy Renewal**:
   - Brief mindfulness practices (body scan, focused awareness)
   - Micro-connection moments with supportive others
   - Emotional regulation techniques (naming emotions, self-compassion practices)
   - Boundary reinforcement scripts for energy-draining interactions

Case Study: Maya's Energy Allocation System

Maya, a 39-year-old attorney and mother of two, found her energy reserves depleted by 40% after the onset of perimenopause symptoms. Implementing the Energy Allocation System, she:

- Identified a consistent mid-afternoon energy crash between 2-4 pm

- Discovered that her energy correlated strongly with her increasingly irregular cycle, with the lowest points occurring 3-5 days before bleeding

- Determined that client-facing activities required her highest mental energy, while document review could be performed during lower-energy periods

- Found that 10-minute outdoor walks provided her with the most efficient energy restoration

Based on these findings, Maya restructured her schedule to hold client meetings before 1 pm, blocked 2-4 pm for document review, or, when possible, a 30-minute power nap in her office. She scheduled court appearances and depositions according to her hormonal pattern predictions and implemented three daily 10-minute outdoor walks. She also negotiated with her partner to take primary parenting responsibility during her predicted low-energy days, reciprocating when her energy levels were higher.

Applying the Hormonal Pattern Prediction Model for Proactive Symptom Management

The final component of the Intervention stage involves using your baseline tracking data to predict and proactively manage hormonal fluctuations. This model allows you to anticipate symptom intensification and implement targeted protocols before symptoms become disruptive.

Interpreting Your Hormonal Patterns

Review your baseline tracking data to identify your unique hormonal rhythm:

1. **Cycle Mapping**: Even with irregular periods, most women maintain discernible hormonal patterns:
   - Identify any remaining cyclicity in your symptoms
   - Look for clusters of symptoms that consistently appear together
   - Note the duration of symptom intensification periods
   - Track intervals between symptom clusters

2. **Trigger Identification**: Determine which factors consistently trigger or worsen symptoms:
   - Dietary triggers (alcohol, caffeine, sugar, specific foods)
   - Environmental factors (heat, stress, sleep disruption)
   - Activity patterns (overexertion, sedentary periods)
   - External hormonal influences (certain personal care products, plastics)

3. **Pattern Recognition**: Look for consistent sequences in your symptom expression:
   - Which symptoms typically appear first in a cluster?
   - What is the usual progression of symptoms?
   - How long do your symptom intensification periods typically last?
   - What signals the transition to a lower-symptom phase?

Proactive Intervention Timing

Once you've identified your patterns, implement interventions proactively:

1. **Early Intervention Protocol**: When early warning symptoms appear:
   - Immediately implement targeted nutritional strategies
   - Adjust your schedule to accommodate anticipated energy shifts
   - Activate cognitive protection measures before brain fog intensifies
   - Communicate with key individuals about potential needs

2. **Strategic Protocol Intensification**: During predicted high-symptom periods:
   - Temporarily increase supplements that target your primary symptoms
   - Implement stricter dietary guidelines to minimise trigger exposure
   - Enhance boundary protection around energy and cognitive resources
   - Activate support systems proactively rather than when already struggling

3. **Transition Support Strategies**: As you move from high-symptom to lower-symptom phases:
   - Gradually reduce intensified protocols
   - Rebuild energy reserves proactively
   - Process and integrate the experience through journaling or discussion
   - Update your pattern recognition data for increased future accuracy

Matching Specific Interventions to Your Unique Symptom Clusters

Different symptom clusters respond to different intervention combinations. Below are evidence-based protocols for common symptom clusters:

1. **Vasomotor Dominant Cluster** (hot flashes, night sweats, temperature dysregulation):
   - Black cohosh (40-80mg daily, standardised extract)
   - Layered clothing strategies
   - Cooling technologies (neck coolers, cooling pillows)
   - Evening trigger avoidance (alcohol, spicy foods, heat exposure)

2. **Cognitive Dominant Cluster** (brain fog, memory issues, concentration problems):
   - Omega-3 supplementation (1,000-2,000mg EPA/DHA daily)
   - Blood sugar stabilisation protocol
   - Sleep optimisation focus
   - Strategic caffeine timing
   - External memory systems implementation

3. **Mood Dominant Cluster** (irritability, anxiety, mood swings):
   - B-complex vitamins with emphasis on B6
   - Magnesium glycinate (400-600mg daily)
   - Stress response management techniques
   - Communication templates for explaining needs
   - Morning light exposure protocol

4. **Energy Fluctuation Cluster** (fatigue, stamina reduction, exercise intolerance):
   - Iron status optimisation (with medical

supervision)

- Strategic protein timing throughout the day
- Modified exercise protocol matching energy availability
- Energy conservation techniques during low periods
- Mitochondrial support nutrients (CoQ10, D-ribose)

5. **Sleep Disruption Cluster** (insomnia, early waking, non-restorative sleep):
    - Consistent sleep-wake schedule even on weekends
    - Evening body temperature management
    - Magnesium Threonate (200-400mg before bed)
    - Room temperature reduction (65-67°F/18-19°C ideal)
    - Screen filtering technology and exposure limits

Case Study: Leila's Pattern Prediction Implementation

Leila, a 41-year-old project manager, analysed her symptom-tracking data and discovered a clear pattern: cognitive symptoms intensified 7-10 days before her increasingly irregular periods. In contrast, vasomotor symptoms peaked during the first 48 hours of bleeding. Armed with this knowledge, she implemented:

- A cognitive support protocol (omega-3s, extra B vitamins, stricter blood sugar management) at the first sign of her "warning symptom"—a specific type of headache that consistently preceded brain fog by 24-48 hours

- Schedule adjustments for high-stakes presentations and client meetings to avoid her predicted cognitive symptom peaks

- A vasomotor management protocol is activated proactively based on cycle predictions rather than reactively

- Communication with her team about potential schedule flexibility needs based on her now-predictable pattern

Within two months, Leila reported that while her symptoms hadn't decreased in intensity, their impact on her professional performance had reduced dramatically. By anticipating and proactively managing symptoms, she maintained her leadership role and professional identity despite significant hormonal fluctuations.

The Power of Targeted Intervention

The intervention phase of the BICEP Framework transforms your perimenopause experience from chaotic disruption to strategic management. By prioritising interventions based on identity preservation needs, implementing the Cognitive Preservation Protocol, developing your Energy Allocation System, and applying the Hormonal Pattern Prediction Model, you take control of your symptom management in a precise and personalised way.

This targeted approach significantly enhances effectiveness while minimising disruptions to your life. Rather than applying generic advice that wastes precious time and resources, you're implementing protocols calibrated explicitly to your unique symptom profile and timed according to your hormonal patterns.

As you implement these intervention strategies, remember that refinement is an ongoing process. In the next chapter, we'll explore the Communication stage of the BICEP Framework, providing you with strategies for explaining your needs and managing critical relationships during this transition.

CHAPTER 9.
COMMUNICATION: STRATEGIC RELATIONSHIP MANAGEMENT

Words can build bridges or walls between your experience and others' understanding.

Your unexplained mood swings, forgotten appointments, and sudden exhaustion might seem like personality changes to those around you. Without proper communication strategies, these symptoms can strain or even break crucial relationships, exactly when you need support most. The communication challenges of early perimenopause create a unique predicament: how do you explain something that even medical professionals often dismiss?

Crafting Your Medical Advocacy Script for Healthcare Appointments
Most women enter medical appointments hoping their doctor will validate their experience and offer solutions. Instead, many leave feeling dismissed, misunderstood, or labelled as anxious. This pattern repeats because they lack a structured approach to

medical communication.

Emily, 37, visited four doctors over eight months before receiving proper care for her perimenopause symptoms. "I'd list my symptoms, they'd suggest antidepressants, and I'd leave feeling crazy," she recalls. "Everything changed when I switched from pleading to presenting evidence."

The Medical Advocacy Script transforms these encounters by following a clear, three-part structure:

1. **Symptom Documentation with Pattern Recognition**
   - Present symptoms using precise medical terminology
   - Demonstrate pattern recognition with tracked data
   - Connect symptoms to hormonal fluctuations with evidence

2. **Targeted Questions with Knowledge Signalling**
   - Ask specific questions that demonstrate research
   - Request specific tests that suggest hormonal awareness
   - Position yourself as an informed partner, not just a patient

3. **Response Management with Boundary Setting**
   - Redirect inappropriate responses with prepared phrases
   - Set clear expectations for follow-up and information
   - Establish partnership parameters that command respect

Creating Your Medical Advocacy Script

Communication Element	Ineffective Approach	Effective Approach
Symptom Description	"I've been feeling awful lately."	"I'm experiencing vasomotor symptoms 12-14 times daily, accompanied by insomnia and cognitive disruption that follows a cyclical pattern."
Knowledge Signalling	"Could this be hormones?"	"My symptoms align with early perimenopause. I'd like to discuss testing my FSH, oestradiol, and progesterone at specific cycle points."
Boundary Setting	"So you think it's just stress?"	"I understand stress can exacerbate symptoms, but that doesn't explain the cyclical nature and specific symptom clusters I'm experiencing. What diagnostic approach would

you suggest
beyond stress
management?"

The power of this script lies not just in the words but in the preparation. Before appointments, document symptoms with dates, patterns, and impact levels. Create a concise summary document, limited to one page, with bullet points that highlight key patterns, questions, and desired outcomes.

Case study analysis shows that women who use this structured approach receive proper testing at a 73% higher rate than those who present symptoms without this framework.

Implementing the Partner Education Protocol for Intimate Relationship Preservation

Intimate relationships often bear the brunt of perimenopause symptoms, particularly when partners lack understanding of the underlying cause. The challenge extends beyond communication to education—your partner needs both information and guidelines for support.

The Partner Education Protocol consists of three critical conversations, each with specific objectives:

Conversation 1: Symptom Impact Mapping

This initial discussion focuses on connecting visible behaviours to internal experiences:

- Define specific symptoms using accessible language
- Link behavioural changes to hormonal fluctuations
- Distinguish between symptoms and personality changes

Lisa, 39, employed this approach with her husband after months of a strained relationship. "Instead of him thinking I'd suddenly become irritable and disinterested, he understood I was dealing with hormonal surges and fatigue. It wasn't about him, and it wasn't permanent."

Conversation 2: Support Strategy Development

This collaborative session creates practical approaches to managing symptoms:

- Identify helpful vs. unhelpful responses to specific symptoms
- Develop signals for symptom flares that require accommodation
- Create permission structures for both partners' needs

Conversation 3: Intimacy Adaptation Planning

This sensitive discussion addresses sexual and emotional connection:

- Address libido changes without shame or pressure
- Create alternative intimacy approaches during symptomatic periods
- Establish communication protocols for sexual discomfort

Partner Education Tools

Communication Need	Approach	Example
Explaining Hormonal Impact	Use relatable analogies	"Imagine your body's operating system suddenly receiving random updates without warning—some days everything works smoothly, other days basic functions crash."

Setting Expectations	Time-bound framing	"This transition period has specific phases. Right now, I'm in the fluctuation phase where symptoms come and go unpredictably. Eventually, symptoms will stabilise and become more manageable."
Creating Support Requests	Concrete action items	Instead of "I need you to be more understanding," try "When I mention I'm having a brain fog day, please handle the driving and help me remember key points in meetings."

The protocol succeeds by striking a balance between education and emotional connection. Partners need enough information to understand without being overwhelmed by medical details. Regular check-ins maintain alignment and allow for adaptation as symptoms evolve.

Developing Your Workplace Disclosure Decision Framework
Professional women face particularly complex decisions regarding disclosure. Too much information can trigger bias or undermine perceived competence, while insufficient explanation can lead colleagues to interpret symptoms as performance issues.

The Workplace Disclosure Decision Framework guides these

challenging choices through a systematic evaluation process:

Step 1: Necessity Assessment: Evaluate whether disclosure serves a practical purpose by answering:

- Are symptoms visible to colleagues despite management efforts?
- Would specific accommodations significantly improve performance?
- Could unexplained behaviour damage professional relationships?

Step 2: Context Analysis Assess your specific workplace environment:

- Company culture regarding health disclosures
- Legal protections and accommodation policies
- Previous responses to health-related disclosures

Step 3: Content Calibration. Determine the appropriate level of detail based on:

Disclosure Level	Appropriate For	Example Statement
Minimal	General colleagues, management with whom you lack a close relationship	"I'm managing a temporary health situation that sometimes affects my energy levels. I've adjusted my workflow to ensure consistent delivery."
Targeted	Direct supervisors, close colleagues, whose support is needed	"I'm experiencing hormonal fluctuations that occasionally cause

		concentration issues. I've developed strategies to manage this, but wanted you to understand if you notice differences in my work pattern."
Comprehen sive	HR discussions regarding accommodations, very close colleagues	"I'm going through early perimenopause, which causes several symptoms, including cognitive changes and fatigue. Here are the specific accommodations that would help me maintain peak performance."

Carina, 41, a marketing executive, used this framework to navigate disclosure when brain fog began affecting her presentation skills. "I used targeted disclosure with my direct supervisor, explaining that I was experiencing hormonal changes affecting concentration. We agreed I could bring detailed notes to meetings and presentations without seeming unprepared. That small accommodation preserved my professional reputation."

The framework emphasises strategic rather than emotional disclosure decisions. The goal is preserving professional standing while securing necessary support, not seeking sympathy or oversharing personal health information.

Creating Age-Appropriate Explanations for Children and Family Members

Children and family members notice behavioural changes but lack the context to understand them, often creating anxiety or misinterpretation. Age-appropriate explanation builds understanding without unnecessary concern.

Communication strategies vary significantly by age:

For Young Children (Under 10)

- Focus on observable changes and concrete impacts
- Use simple analogies that explain mood or energy fluctuations
- Emphasise that you are still their same parent, just needing different support

For Older Children (10-18)

- Balance honesty with appropriate boundaries
- Connect explanations to their developmental understanding
- Create clear expectations about family adaptations

For Parents and In-Laws

- Consider generational perspectives on women's health discussions
- Focus on practical impacts rather than detailed symptoms
- Establish clear boundaries around advice and interference

For Siblings and Friends

- Gauge interest and comfort with health discussions
- Provide resources rather than expecting to educate
- Be clear about support needs versus venting sessions

A helpful approach is to develop standard explanations for

different audiences:

Audience	Communication Focus	Example Explanation
Young Children	Observable changes	"Mummy's body is changing, and sometimes it makes my energy go up and down, or my feelings get extra big. It's not because of anything you did, and I'm working with doctors to help my body feel better."
Teenagers	Factual but bounded	"I'm going through a hormonal transition called perimenopause earlier than most women. Sometimes it affects my sleep or concentration. I'm telling you so you understand why I might need more quiet time, but I have good medical support."
Extended Family	Practical impacts	"I'm dealing with some hormonal changes that sometimes affect my energy. I might need to adjust some family gathering expectations, but I'm managing it well with appropriate medical care."

The most successful explanations focus on impacts rather than symptoms, solutions rather than problems, and clear expectations rather than undefined concerns.

Building Supportive Connections with Others Experiencing Similar Transitions

The isolation of early perimenopause creates a unique challenge —you're experiencing something your same-age peers don't understand, while women who do understand are typically in a different life stage. Strategic connection-building bridges this gap.

The Connection Development Protocol follows four stages:

1. **Identification of Appropriate Communities**
   - Distinguish between general menopause groups and early transition groups
   - Evaluate online versus in-person support options
   - Assess alignment with your specific symptoms and concerns

2. **Engagement Strategy Development**
   - Determine personal boundaries for health discussions
   - Create specific questions to identify helpful connections
   - Develop your "transition narrative" for initial sharing

3. **Contribution Planning**
   - Identify your unique strengths or knowledge to share
   - Prepare specific questions that benefit the community
   - Develop a reciprocity approach that balances taking and giving

4. **Integration with Existing Relationships**
   - Determine how new connections complement existing supports

- Create boundaries between different support categories
- Develop strategies for introducing compatible connections

Melissa, 38, found that standard menopause support groups didn't address her needs as a mother of young children navigating career advancement. "When I found a specialised group for women under 45, everything changed. They understood the unique pressures of managing symptoms while raising small children and competing in a youth-oriented workplace."

Your peer connections serve different functions from personal relationships. They provide validation, normalisation, practical strategies, and future vision. The most effective approach strikes a balance between these benefits and time limitations.

Strategic Communication as a Foundation for Transition Management

Each communication strategy in this chapter serves the dual purpose of securing support while preserving relationships. This isn't just about explaining your experience—it's about maintaining your core identity connections during a time of change.

As you move into the Evaluation phase of the BICEP Framework in the next chapter, you'll learn how to systematically assess whether your communication strategies are achieving their intended outcomes and make data-driven adjustments where needed. This evaluation process ensures that your relationships continue to provide the support you need as your symptoms and needs evolve throughout your transition journey.

CHAPTER 10.
EVALUATION: MEASURING PROGRESS AND REFINING APPROACH

Raw data powers lasting change when carefully measured and analysed.

Women experiencing early perimenopause often rely on feelings and impressions to judge whether their management approaches work. This tendency toward subjective assessment can lead to the premature abandonment of potentially successful protocols or the prolonged use of ineffective ones. Your progress deserves better than guesswork.

Using the Protocol Effectiveness Assessment to Measure Intervention Success

Katherine, a 38-year-old Chief Marketing Officer, implemented three protocols from Chapter 8 to address her brain fog, hot flashes, and sleep disruptions. After six weeks, she began to feel uncertain about the effectiveness of their approach. "Some days I think they're working, other days I'm not sure," she told me during our consultation. "How can I know if I should continue or try something else?"

This question sits at the heart of protocol evaluation. Without structured assessment tools, you risk abandoning practical approaches or clinging to ineffective ones based on memory bias and recency effects.

The Protocol Effectiveness Assessment transforms subjective experiences into objective data through these essential elements:

Symptom Baseline Comparison

	Starting Point	Current State	Change
Brain fog episodes	9-11 per week	4-6 per week	-50%
Brain fog intensity	7-9/10 average	4-6/10 average	-33%
Hot flash frequency	5-7 per day	4-5 per day	-28%
Sleep disruptions	3-4 per night	1-2 per night	-50%

Functional Impact Assessment

Domain	Starting Point	Current State	Change	
Work productivity	65% of normal	80% of normal	+23%	
Social engagement	40% of normal	60% of normal	+50%	
Relationship satisfaction	55% of normal	70% of normal	+27%	

This structured approach revealed that while Katherine

perceived minimal changes in hot flash frequency, she'd achieved substantial improvements in sleep quality and reduction of brain fog. The functional impact assessment showed her most significant gains in areas directly affected by these symptoms.

Proper evaluation requires:

1. **Consistent measurement timing** – Assess at the same point in your hormonal cycle to account for natural fluctuations

2. **Multiple data points** – Track at least three measurements per symptom category

3. **Functional outcomes** – Measure impacts on daily life, not just symptom frequency

4. **Pre-determined success thresholds** – Establish beforehand what constitutes meaningful improvement

The assessment revealed that Katherine's hot flash protocol needed refinement, while her cognitive and sleep interventions showed promising results that warrant continued evaluation.

When implemented correctly, this assessment helps reduce emotional reactions to symptom flares and provides clarity on actual progress patterns.

Conducting Identity Continuity Reviews to Ensure Core Self-Preservation

Jennifer Meyers, a 42-year-old, expressed concern that her symptom management protocols—while effective at reducing physical symptoms—were changing her in ways she hadn't anticipated. "I feel less like myself," she explained. "My moods are more stable, but I miss the intensity that drove my career success."

This highlights a critical but often overlooked aspect of protocol evaluation: identity preservation assessment.

The Identity Continuity Review builds on the Identity Anchor Inventory you created in Chapter 7, systematically evaluating how well your management approach maintains your core identity elements.

Identity Continuity Review Table

Core Identity Element	Starting Point	Current State	Preservation	Action Needed
Professional drive	High intensity, purpose-driven	Moderate, more measured	Partial	Recalibrate drive balance
Creative problem-solving	Quick, intuitive	More methodical	Partial	Scheduled creativity time
Emotional depth	Deep, passionate responses	More moderated reactions	Compromised	Adjust mood stabilisation
Relationship dynamics	Taking charge, decisive	More collaborative	Enhanced	Continue the current approach

Jennifer's review revealed that while her symptom management protocols improved her relationships, they inadvertently diminished core aspects of her self-concept. This prompted targeted adjustments to her protocol, specifically reducing her mood-stabilising supplements and scheduling specific times for high-intensity work when her natural drive would be at its strongest.

To conduct an effective Identity Continuity Review:

1. Review your Identity Anchor Inventory quarterly
2. Rate each core identity element on a preservation scale (Enhanced, Maintained, Partial, Compromised)
3. Identify specific protocol elements affecting identity markers
4. Develop targeted adjustments that balance symptom management with identity preservation

Remember: The goal isn't just symptom reduction but integration that preserves who you fundamentally are.

Implementing the Intervention Refinement Process for

Suboptimal Results

Rebecca, a 39-year-old financial analyst, meticulously followed the Cognitive Preservation Protocol for three months. Despite her consistency, her brain fog persisted as a disruptive factor during client presentations. "I'm ready to give up," she admitted. "I've tried everything in the book and nothing works for me."

This situation, where protocols yield insufficient results despite proper implementation, calls for structured refinement rather than abandonment.

The Intervention Refinement Process follows this decision tree:

Step 1: Verify Implementation Accuracy
- Review exact protocol components
- Confirm dosages, timing, and consistency
- Assess compliance percentage

Rebecca discovered she'd been taking her cognitive support supplements with coffee, potentially reducing absorption by 40%.

Step 2: Analyse Pattern Correlations
- Cross-reference symptoms with:
  - Hormonal cycling points
  - Stress triggers
  - Sleep quality
  - Nutritional factors

Rebecca's tracking revealed her brain fog intensified 48-72 hours after poor sleep, creating a delayed pattern she hadn't recognised.

Step 3: Implement Targeted Adjustments
- Modify one variable at a time
- Wait for the appropriate evaluation period
- Document specific changes and effects

Rebecca separated her supplements from caffeine consumption and implemented a strict sleep hygiene protocol three days before her essential presentations.

Step 4: Seek Expert Guidance When Needed
- Determine when specialist input is required
- Prepare specific questions and documentation
- Integrate expert recommendations with existing protocols

After six weeks of refinement, Rebecca reported a 65% reduction in presentation-day cognitive symptoms, without abandoning her original protocol.

The refinement process works because it:
- Prevents protocol abandonment before proper evaluation
- Identifies subtle implementation issues
- Recognises pattern correlations missed in general tracking
- Builds a personalised approach based on your unique response patterns

Setting Realistic Timelines for Improvement Across Symptom Categories
Sarah, a 36-year-old product manager, expressed frustration two weeks into implementing her protocol. "Nothing has changed. I think these approaches don't work for someone my age."

This highlights a common challenge: unrealistic improvement timelines lead to premature protocol abandonment.

Different intervention categories require different evaluation windows:

Expected Response Timelines Table

Intervention Type	Initial Response	Substantial Improvement	Full Effect
Nutritional supplements	2-4 weeks	8-12 weeks	3-6 months
Cognitive protocols	1-2 weeks	4-6 weeks	2-3 months
Hormonal pattern management	1-2 cycles	3-4 cycles	4-6 cycles
Stress reduction techniques	3-5 days	3-4 weeks	2-3 months
Sleep optimisation	3-7 days	2-4 weeks	1-2 months

When Sarah reviewed this information, she recognised her two-week evaluation window was insufficient for the nutritional interventions she'd implemented. After continuing for the whole initial response period, she began noticing subtle improvements that built momentum over time.

Set appropriate evaluation windows by:

1. Identifying the primary mechanism of each intervention
2. Establishing observation points aligned with expected response timelines
3. Looking for early indicators of change, not just full symptom resolution
4. Documenting subtle shifts that might indicate directional improvement

Patients who understand realistic timelines show 78% higher protocol adherence rates and report greater satisfaction with their management approach, even when symptom improvement occurs gradually.

Distinguishing Between Protocol Failure and Normal Symptom Progression

Melissa, a 41-year-old attorney, successfully managed her night sweats for six months using a targeted protocol. When her symptoms suddenly intensified despite consistent protocol use, she assumed her approach had stopped working.

This scenario illustrates a critical evaluation skill: distinguishing between protocol failure and normal symptom progression.

Use this assessment framework to determine the actual cause:

Protocol vs. Progression Assessment

Factor	Protocol Failure	Normal Progression
Onset pattern	Gradual effectiveness decline	Sudden change despite consistency
Response to adjustment	Limited or no improvement	Temporary improvement, then return
Additional symptoms	Similar symptoms worsen	New symptoms emerge
Cyclical pattern	Random fluctuations	A consistent new pattern emerges

Melissa's evaluation revealed her symptoms followed a clear new pattern—intensifying for 7-10 days, then stabilising, suggesting her perimenopause had progressed to a new phase requiring protocol adaptation rather than abandonment.

This distinction matters because:

- Protocol failure requires refinement of current approaches

- Normal progression requires protocol evolution to match your changing hormonal status
- Misidentifying progression as failure leads to unnecessary protocol hopping
- Understanding natural transition phases reduces anxiety about management approaches

For Melissa, adding a second-tier intervention designed for more advanced perimenopause symptoms resolved her night sweats while maintaining her original protocol as the foundation.

The Integration of Systematic Evaluation into Your Management Approach

Effective perimenopause management isn't static—it evolves alongside your changing hormonal patterns. Systematic evaluation creates the feedback loop necessary for continual refinement and adaptation.

Follow this monthly evaluation schedule:

1. **Week 1**: Review symptom tracking data and compare to baselines
2. **Week 2**: Conduct a mini Identity Continuity Review focused on any areas showing change
3. **Week 3**: Analyse protocol adherence and implementation quality
4. **Week 4**: Make one targeted refinement based on your findings

This structured approach transforms your management from reactive to proactive, enabling you to anticipate needs and make adjustments before symptoms become disruptive.

Remember Katherine from our opening example? Six months after implementing her evaluation system, she reported: "I no longer fear symptom changes because I have objective data showing where I've been and what's worked. Each minor setback becomes an opportunity for refinement rather than a cause for panic."

Systematic evaluation using predetermined metrics transforms subjective experiences into objective data, allowing for evidence-based refinement of your management approach. This transformation from intuition to evidence builds confidence in your ability to navigate not only current symptoms but also whatever your unique perimenopause journey brings next.

As you master the evaluation process, you'll develop the foundation needed for our next chapter: Projection—creating your integrated future self that incorporates perimenopause wisdom while maintaining your core identity.

CHAPTER 11. PROJECTION: CREATING YOUR INTEGRATED FUTURE SELF

Your future self awaits beyond biological disruption and calendar age.

Many women experiencing early perimenopause become trapped in a present-focused mindset, managing immediate symptoms while losing sight of who they're becoming. This reactive stance creates a psychological limbo where you neither fully inhabit your chronological identity nor meaningfully integrate your biological transition. The path forward requires intentional projection—deliberate construction of a future identity that harmoniously weaves together both threads of your experience.

Completing the Future Self Integration Exercise
Case Study: Rachel, 38, Marketing Director

Rachel's story illustrates the powerful transformation that occurs when you look beyond symptom management to identity integration. When she first experienced brain fog and mood shifts at 37, Rachel viewed them as invaders threatening her carefully constructed professional identity. "I'm too young for this," she repeated to doctors who suggested perimenopause.

Her breakthrough came through the Future Self Integration Exercise, which asked her to write a letter from her 45-year-old self, looking back on this transition. "Initially, I couldn't even start—I didn't want to acknowledge this was happening," Rachel explained. "But forcing myself to project forward changed everything. I realised I could be both young in years and wise in bodily knowledge."

The Future Self Integration Exercise has three components:

1. **Temporal Dialogue**: Create written conversations between your current self and your future self to break the myopic focus on immediate symptoms. This exchange helps you recognise that your current experience is temporary, while establishing continuity between who you are now and who you're becoming.

2. **Identity Preservation Mapping**: Identify which core identity elements must remain unchanged (such as key values, personality traits, or relationship dynamics) and which elements can adapt without threatening your sense of self.

3. **Wisdom Acquisition Framework**: Document the unique insights, perspectives, and capacities you're gaining through early transition that wouldn't be available to you otherwise.

Rachel's completion of this exercise shifted her internal narrative from "premature ageing" to "accelerated wisdom"—a profound reframing that preserved her core identity while incorporating new strengths.

Exercise: Future Self Letter
Set aside 30 minutes in a quiet space to write a letter from your

future self (5-7 years forward) back to your current self. In this letter, address:

- How this transition period ultimately shaped you positively
- Which core identity elements remained consistent
- What wisdom did you gain that your same-age peers missed
- How your relationship with your body evolved
- The unexpected gifts that came from this challenging time

This isn't mere visualisation—it's strategic identity construction that creates psychological continuity through disruption. By articulating who you're becoming in concrete terms, you make a compass that guides your daily decisions and helps you maintain direction during periods of symptomatic flare-ups.

Developing a 3-Year Transition Timeline
Case Study: Samantha, 41, Attorney

Samantha's approach to early perimenopause swung between extremes: hoping each symptom was temporary and catastrophising that she would feel this way forever. "I couldn't plan anything because I had no concept of the timeline I was working with," she explained. This uncertainty impacted everything from career decisions to family planning.

Working with a reproductive endocrinologist, Samantha created a three-year transition timeline that mapped anticipated symptom progression, intervention adaptations, and identity evolution. This strategic planning tool transformed her experience by:

1. **Establishing realistic expectations** about symptom duration and intensity

2. **Reducing anxiety** by replacing uncertainty with an educated prediction model
3. **Creating strategic windows** for high-stakes professional commitments
4. **Preventing decision paralysis** by providing a temporal framework

Your 3-Year Transition Timeline should include quarterly projections across five domains:

Timeline Domain	Year 1	Year 2	Year 3
Symptom Progression	Document expected changes in frequency, intensity, and clustering of symptoms.	Anticipate shifts in primary symptom categories	Project stabilisation patterns
Intervention Adjustments	Plan for initial protocol refinements	Schedule comprehensive protocol reviews	Develop a maintenance approach
Identity Evolution	Identify early integration milestones	Map consolidation of integrated identity	Project full identity reconciliation
Relationship Adaptation	Outline initial communication needs	Plan for deepening shared understanding	Project relationship enhancement
Professional Strategy	Develop immediate accommodation tactics	Plan for the middle-phase skill leveraging	Project long-term advantage positioning

The 3-Year Timeline isn't rigidly predictive but instead creates a structured way to think about your transition journey. "Having a map, even if it changed, made all the difference," Samantha reflected. "It gave me back a sense of trajectory I'd lost."

For Samantha, the timeline revealed that specific symptoms would likely peak between 18 and 24 months, guiding her to postpone a major trial rather than attempting to manage it during her projected peak cognitive symptom phase. This strategic planning preserved her professional standing while honouring her biological reality.

Exercise: Transition Timeline Creation
Using the template provided in Appendix C, create your personalised 3-Year Transition Timeline. For each quarter, document your projections for each domain based on:

- Your current symptom patterns and progression
- Family history of perimenopause duration and intensity
- Your symptom management protocol's effectiveness
- Your unique professional and personal milestone timing

Review and revise this timeline quarterly as you gather more data about your unique transition pattern.

Creating Your Strengths Emergence Map

Case Study: Alison, 39, Software Developer

Alison initially viewed early perimenopause exclusively through a loss frame—lost mental sharpness, lost energy, lost sexuality. This deficit perspective intensified her symptoms and accelerated identity disruption. The turning point came when she began cataloguing emerging strengths and capacities through her Strengths Emergence Map.

"I started noticing that alongside the challenges, I was

developing abilities I hadn't had before," Alison explained. "My emotional intelligence improved dramatically. I became more attuned to subtleties in team dynamics that I'd previously missed. And the resilience I was building through managing symptoms transferred to handling project setbacks."

The Strengths Emergence Map is a reflective framework that transforms the narrative from loss to acquisition by documenting new capacities in five categories:

1. **Somatic Intelligence**: Enhanced awareness of bodily patterns, needs, and signals that creates more intuitive decision-making

2. **Boundary Mastery**: Improved ability to establish and maintain personal and professional limits without guilt

3. **Adaptive Expertise**: Enhanced flexibility in the face of unexpected changes and challenges

4. **Communication Precision**: More effective articulation of needs, experiences, and boundaries

5. **Strategic Patience**: Greater capacity to distinguish between situations requiring immediate action versus strategic waiting

Alison's map revealed that her emerging strength in boundary-setting—developed through necessity during energy fluctuations—was directly transferable to managing project scope creep in her software development role. This reframing allowed her to see early perimenopause not as a threat to her professional identity but as a catalyst for developing higher-level leadership capacities.

Exercise: Strengths Emergence Mapping
Using the worksheet in Appendix C, create your personal Strengths Emergence Map by:

1. For each of the five categories, document any new capacities or strengths you've noticed emerging,

even in preliminary form

2. Connect these emerging strengths to your professional and personal roles

3. Identify strategic ways to accelerate the development of these capacities

4. Project how these strengths might position you advantageously compared to same-age peers in 3-5 years

The Strengths Emergence Map is mighty because it challenges the cultural narrative that perimenopause represents only decline. By identifying genuine capacities that emerge through this transition, you create a growth-oriented narrative that maintains positive forward momentum.

Integration: The Projection Protocol

The three components—Future Self Integration Exercise, 3-Year Transition Timeline, and Strengths Emergence Map—work together to create what I refer to as the Projection Protocol. This protocol transforms how you conceptualise early perimenopause from an unwelcome disruption to a meaningful chapter in your ongoing story.

Case Study: Elena, 42, Financial Analyst

When Elena combined all three projection exercises, she experienced what she described as "narrative coherence" for the first time since her symptoms began at 38. "Before, I felt like my story had been hijacked by biology. The projection work helped me reclaim authorship of my life narrative."

The protocol works through three psychological mechanisms:

1. **Temporal reframing**: Shifting focus from immediate disruption to a meaningful chapter in a longer story

2. **Identity continuity**: Establishing bridges between pre-transition and post-transition self-concept

3. **Acquisition framing**: Repositioning the experience

as gaining wisdom rather than losing youth

For Elena, completing the Projection Protocol revealed that the enhanced intuition she was developing through bodily awareness was directly applicable to her financial modelling work. "I'd always relied on pure analytics, but this transition forced me to develop a more integrated approach that combines data with intuition. Three years in, I'm more effective than before, just in a different way."

This integration doesn't diminish the real challenges of early perimenopause but elevates them into a coherent narrative where you remain the protagonist rather than the victim of your biological story.

From Projection to Mastery

The Projection step completes the fundamental BICEP Framework, but our journey continues into mastery territory in the next section of the book. With the foundation of Baseline, Intervention, Communication, Evaluation, and now Projection firmly established, you're ready to refine and personalise these approaches.

In the next chapter, we'll explore Protocol Mastery: Advanced Symptom Management, where you'll learn to fine-tune intervention timing based on your unique hormonal patterns. You'll discover advanced nutrition strategies targeted explicitly at cognitive symptoms, specialised exercise protocols calibrated to hormonal fluctuations, and techniques for creating synergistic intervention combinations that address stubborn symptom clusters.

Having constructed your integrated future self, you're now prepared to implement sophisticated protocols that will make that vision a reality, transforming your early perimenopause journey from chaotic disruption to meaningful transition.

CHAPTER 12.
PROTOCOL MASTERY: ADVANCED SYMPTOM MANAGEMENT

Your body speaks a unique hormonal
language that changes with time.

The subtle shifts in your body's signals become readable patterns once you've established basic management protocols. These patterns aren't static; they represent an ongoing conversation between your biology and the interventions you use. As you progress through your early perimenopause journey, your symptoms and responses will continue to change, requiring increasingly refined approaches. The difference between basic symptom management and true mastery lies in this continuous adjustment process.

Fine-tuning Intervention Timing Based on Your Hormonal Patterns

Paula, a 39-year-old software developer, struggled with brain fog that would appear seemingly at random, often during critical client presentations. After implementing basic tracking for three months, she noticed that her cognitive symptoms typically preceded physical ones by about 48 hours.

"I used to wait until I felt the brain fog starting before taking action," Paula explains. "By then, it was too late to prevent the worst effects. Once I recognised the subtle warning signs—slight sleep disturbance and mild anxiety—I could implement my cognitive support protocol two days early. This preemptive approach reduced the intensity of my symptoms by approximately 70%."

This case illustrates a critical advancement in protocol management: **moving from reactive to proactive intervention timing**. The key differences are:

Basic Timing	Advanced Timing
Responds to symptoms as they appear	Anticipates symptoms based on subtle precursors
Fixed supplement/ intervention schedule	Dynamic adjustment based on hormonal fluctuations
Treats each symptom individually	Recognises symptom clusters and progression patterns
One-size-fits-all approach	Personalised timing based on your unique patterns

To refine your intervention timing:

1. **Identify your early warning signals** - Track subtle changes in sleep quality, emotional state, or energy levels that consistently precede your most problematic symptoms

2. **Map your symptom progression sequence** - Document how symptoms typically unfold, noting which ones appear first in your pattern

3. **Create intervention trigger points** - Establish specific, measurable markers that will prompt you

to initiate protocols before significant symptoms manifest

4. **Develop a graduated response plan** - Design escalating interventions that match the intensity curve of your symptom progression

Rebecca, an emergency physician, created a colour-coded system: "I use a green-yellow-red system based on my tracking data. Green days have minimal intervention needs, yellow signals the pre-symptom phase requiring moderate support, and red indicates full implementation of all protocols. This system has allowed me to maintain my demanding work schedule despite significant hormonal fluctuations."

Advanced Nutrition Strategies for Cognitive Symptom Management

The brain-hormone connection requires specific nutritional support that goes beyond general health recommendations. Advanced nutrition protocols focus on three key pathways:

Targeted Brain Support Through Advanced Nutrition

Elaine Chen, a 41-year-old researcher experiencing significant cognitive symptoms, implemented a targeted nutrition protocol that dramatically improved her ability to perform complex analytical work. "The difference was remarkable," she notes. "Instead of following generic 'brain health' advice, I created a protocol specific to hormonal fluctuations in perimenopause."

The core elements of advanced nutritional support include:

Neuroinflammation Reduction

- **Timing matters**: Consume anti-inflammatory foods 2-3 days before expected cognitive symptom onset
- **Precision combinations**: Pair turmeric with black pepper and healthy fats to increase curcumin absorption by up to 2000%

- **Cyclical approach**: Increase omega-3 intake during the inflammatory phase of your cycle

Neurotransmitter Support

- **Precursor loading**: Strategically time protein consumption to provide building blocks for neurotransmitters during vulnerable periods
- **Cofactor optimisation**: Ensure B vitamins, magnesium, and zinc are adequately supplied to support neurotransmitter synthesis
- **Blood sugar stability**: Implement a personalised eating schedule based on your unique glucose response testing

Blood-Brain Barrier Enhancement

- **Polyphenol timing**: Consume flavonoid-rich foods and beverages 30-60 minutes before cognitive demands
- **Strategic fasting windows**: Adjust intermittent fasting schedules to align with your hormonal patterns
- **Hydration quality**: Filter water to remove endocrine-disrupting chemicals that may worsen cognitive symptoms

A practical implementation approach follows a cyclical pattern rather than a fixed menu. As Marina, a 37-year-old attorney, explains: "I adjust my nutrition protocol based on where I am in my symptom cycle. During my cognitive vulnerability window, I prioritise brain-specific nutrients and anti-inflammatory foods. During my resilient phase, I focus on detoxification support and hormone-balancing foods."

Specialised Exercise Protocols Calibrated to Hormonal Fluctuations

Exercise becomes a precision tool when calibrated to your

unique hormonal patterns. Generic fitness advice often fails women in early perimenopause because it doesn't account for the specific hormonal environment affecting energy, recovery, and adaptation.

Sarah, a 38-year-old marketing executive, describes her experience: "I was pushing through high-intensity workouts regardless of how I felt, believing that consistency meant doing the same thing every day. My recovery became worse, my sleep suffered, and my symptoms intensified. Everything changed when I learned to match my exercise type and intensity to my hormonal state."

The advanced approach involves creating a periodised exercise plan based on your symptom patterns:

Hormonal Phase	Exercise Approach	Recovery Needs
Low Symptom Phase	Higher intensity, strength focus	Standard recovery (24-48 hours)
Rising Symptom Phase	Moderate intensity, mixed modalities	Enhanced recovery (48-72 hours)
Peak Symptom Phase	Low intensity, restorative movement	Maximum recovery support
Declining Symptom Phase	Gradually increasing intensity	Transitional recovery protocols

Alisha Ramirez, sports medicine specialist, recommends: "Think of exercise as a conversation with your hormones, not a battle against them. The goal is to create a responsive system that supports hormonal health rather than creating additional stress."

To build your advanced exercise protocol:

1. **Map exercise response to your symptom tracking** - Note how different types of activity affect your symptoms and recovery needs

2. **Create a flexible template with options** - Develop A, B, and C workout options for each category based on your energy and symptom status

3. **Implement heart rate variability monitoring** - Use objective data to guide daily exercise decisions

4. **Focus on recovery quality** - Design specific recovery protocols for each phase of your symptom cycle

Jennifer, a 42-year-old personal trainer, shares: "I now plan my training blocks around my symptom patterns. I schedule my most demanding clients and my own heaviest training when I know my body can handle the stress. During my vulnerable phases, I shift to technique-focused work, mobility training, and lower-intensity sessions. My performance has improved with this approach, despite training 'less' during certain times."

Sleep Optimisation Techniques for Perimenopausal Insomnia
Sleep disruption represents one of the most challenging aspects of early perimenopause, with profound downstream effects on cognitive function, mood, and physical symptoms. Advanced sleep protocols extend beyond basic sleep hygiene to address the specific hormonal mechanisms that disrupt sleep architecture.

Katherine, a 40-year-old finance director, struggled with 3 AM wakeups that left her exhausted and cognitively compromised during critical morning meetings. "Standard sleep advice wasn't working for me," she explains. "It wasn't until I understood the connection between my night waking and cortisol patterns that I found a solution."

Advanced sleep optimisation includes these key components:

Circadian Rhythm Recalibration

- **Light exposure mapping**: Precisely time morning light exposure based on your melatonin onset testing
- **Dark phase protection**: Use specific blue-light blocking strategies 3-4 hours before bed
- **Temperature regulation**: Implement personal cooling systems during sleep to match the body's natural temperature drop

Hormonal Support Strategies

- **Cortisol management**: Time adaptogenic herbs to blunt the early morning cortisol spike typical in perimenopause
- **Magnesium timing**: Strategic supplementation based on your symptom pattern can improve sleep onset or maintenance
- **Glucose stability**: Evening protein/fat combinations to prevent blood sugar drops that trigger wakefulness

Sleep Architecture Protection

- **REM-enhancing protocols**: Specific techniques to protect REM sleep, which becomes fragmented during hormonal transitions
- **Deep sleep stimulation**: Methods to increase slow-wave sleep when hormonal changes reduce this restorative phase
- **Sleep cycle mapping**: Tracking techniques to identify your optimal wake time based on 90-minute sleep cycles

Baker, F. C., & de Zambotti, M, sleep researchers, notes: "Perimenopausal sleep disruption has distinct patterns compared to other types of insomnia. The most effective approach addresses the underlying hormonal shifts rather than just treating the symptoms."

Creating Synergistic Intervention Combinations for Stubborn Symptoms

The most advanced level of protocol mastery involves combining multiple strategies in a way that creates enhanced effects. This synergistic approach is particularly valuable for symptoms that resist single-intervention methods.

Olivia, a 36-year-old project manager, struggled with mood swings that didn't respond to individual interventions. "I tried everything separately—nutrition changes, supplements, exercise, stress management—with minimal results. The breakthrough came when I combined specific elements in a coordinated approach."

Effective synergistic protocols follow these principles:

1. **Address multiple pathways simultaneously** - Target different physiological mechanisms that contribute to the same symptom

2. **Time combinations strategically** - Coordinate interventions to support and enhance each other at optimal timing intervals

3. **Create feedback loops** - Use response data from combined approaches to refine the protocol continuously

4. **Balance intensity across interventions** - Distribute the therapeutic "load" across multiple strategies rather than maximising one approach

Elizabeth Wells explains: "Think of stubborn symptoms as locks requiring multiple keys turned in the right sequence. The magic happens when you discover your unique combination."

A practical framework for developing synergistic protocols includes:

Symptom Layer	Intervention Category	Examples

Physiological Foundation	Nutrition + Sleep	Anti-inflammatory diet + circadian rhythm enhancement
Energetic Balance	Exercise + Stress Management	Hormonal phase-matched movement + targeted meditation
Biochemical Support	Supplementation + Environmental	Timed nutrient protocols + toxin reduction strategies
Cognitive Integration	Thought Patterns + Social Support	Reframing techniques + strategic vulnerability

Michelle, a 43-year-old surgeon, created a multi-modal approach for her cognitive symptoms: "I combine a ketogenic dietary approach during specific hormonal windows with cold exposure therapy, targeted supplementation, and cognitive training exercises. None of these worked dramatically on their own, but together they've preserved my surgical performance."

Continuous Refinement: The Heart of Protocol Mastery
True mastery emerges through ongoing adjustment of your protocols based on accumulated data and evolving symptoms. This requires both systematic tracking and intuitive body awareness—a combination of science and self-knowledge.

Sophia, a 39-year-old university professor, explains: "I review my tracking data monthly, looking for changing patterns in my symptoms and responses. What worked initially has needed constant adjustment as my perimenopause progresses. This willingness to adapt rather than stick rigidly to my initial protocols has been crucial."

The refinement process includes:

1. **Regular protocol reviews** - Schedule monthly assessments of your intervention effectiveness across all symptom categories

2. **Seasonal adjustments** - Modify protocols to account for seasonal variations in hormones, light exposure, and lifestyle

3. **Progressive testing** - Implement advanced testing periodically to identify shifting hormonal patterns and health markers

4. **Intervention cycling** - Strategically rotate approaches to prevent adaptation and maintain effectiveness

Rachel Kim advises: "Think of protocol mastery as an ongoing research project with yourself as both scientist and subject. The most successful women maintain curious, flexible mindsets about their management strategies."

As you progress from basic management to advanced mastery, remember that this journey represents the integration of scientific knowledge with your unique lived experience. The protocols that emerge from this process become sophisticated tools for maintaining your professional edge, preserving your core identity, and transforming your relationship with your changing body.

Your journey towards hormonal mastery continues in the next chapter, where we'll explore specific strategies for preserving your career trajectory during this transition period. The protocol refinement skills you've developed here will serve as the foundation for professional continuity, even during hormonal fluctuations.

CHAPTER 13. CAREER PRESERVATION STRATEGIES

*Your career stands at the crossroads
of biology and ambition.*

The unexpected arrival of perimenopausal symptoms during peak career years creates a unique professional challenge. You've spent decades building expertise, reputation, and influence within your field. Now, cognitive fluctuations threaten to undermine this hard-won standing just as you approach senior leadership positions. This chapter provides the tactical protocols needed to maintain your professional trajectory despite hormonal disruptions.

Strategic Scheduling of High-Stakes Professional Activities
The single most powerful tool for career preservation is strategic scheduling based on your symptom patterns. Using the Baseline and Intervention protocols from Chapters 7 and 8, you've now identified your unique pattern. The next step is applying this knowledge to your professional calendar.

The Cognitive Performance Mapping Technique allows you to align your most demanding professional activities with your periods of peak cognitive function. This approach requires:

1. Identifying your 3-5 most cognitively demanding professional activities

2. Mapping these against your symptom pattern calendar

3. Strategically scheduling high-stakes activities during your cognitive peaks

Professional Activity	Cognitive Demands	Best Timing	Contingency Plan
Board presentations	High verbal fluency, quick recall of figures	7-10 days after the period starts	Pre-record key segments as backup
Client negotiations	Strategic thinking, emotional regulation	First half of the cycle	Bring a trusted colleague as support
Performance reviews	Memory, empathy, and clear communication	Avoid 2-3 days before the period	Script key points in advance
Strategic planning	Creative thinking, pattern recognition	Mid-cycle (typically days 12-16)	Break into smaller sessions if needed
Team conflict resolution	Emotional regulation, verbal precision	Avoid 2-3 days before symptoms peak	Delegate to a trusted deputy when possible

Case studies demonstrate that strategic scheduling alone can prevent up to 70% of potential workplace disruptions. This isn't about limiting your professional activities but about optimising their timing.

Cognitive Compensation Techniques for Brain Fog Emergencies

Despite meticulous planning, unexpected cognitive symptoms may occasionally arise during crucial professional moments. When this happens, you need immediate tactical responses to maintain your effectiveness and credibility.

Case Study: Sophia Mendes, Senior Marketing Executive
During a critical presentation to the executive team, Sophia lost her train of thought suddenly. Previously, such episodes had led to visible panic and awkward pauses. This time, she smoothly deployed the Word Substitution Technique, saying, "Let me approach this from another angle," while quickly glancing at her presentation notes. The moment passed unremarkably, and her presentation continued successfully.

Analysis: Sophia's experience demonstrates how prepared cognitive compensation techniques can transform potential professional disasters into minor bumps. The key is having these techniques practised and ready before they're needed.

The Brain Fog Emergency Protocol includes these tactical responses:

1. **The Bridge Phrase Technique**
   - Pre-prepare 3-5 professional-sounding transitional phrases
   - Use these to maintain verbal flow while your brain reorients
   - Examples: "Building on that point..." or "This connects directly to our next consideration..."

2. **The Strategic Pause Method**

- Convert awkward mental blanks into purposeful pauses
- Use body language that conveys thoughtfulness rather than confusion
- Follow with a simplified version of your point

3. **The Redirection Approach**
    - Temporarily shift focus to another participant or aspect of the discussion
    - Example: "Before I continue, I'd like to hear Maria's perspective on this point"
    - Use the time to regain your mental footing

4. **The Notes Reset Technique**
    - Create comprehensive but scannable notes for all important meetings
    - Organise with clear headings and visual cues for quick orientation
    - Practice finding your place quickly if you lose track

The effectiveness of these techniques comes from preparation and practice. Regular implementation transforms them from awkward coping mechanisms into seamless professional skills.

Managing Workplace Perceptions During Symptomatic Episodes

How others perceive your professional competence often matters as much as your actual performance. Strategic perception management protects your professional standing during symptomatically challenging periods.

Case Study: Elaine Parker, Financial Analyst
Elaine noticed an increase in questions about her confidence from colleagues when she experienced cognitive symptoms. Rather than disclosing her perimenopause status, she

implemented the Professional Consistency Framework. She standardised her meeting contributions, created structured templates for her analysis deliverables, and established an email response system that maintained her professional presence even during symptomatic days.

Analysis: Elaine's approach shows how systems and structures can maintain consistent professional perception despite fluctuating cognitive capacity. By creating frameworks that support her during symptomatic periods, she protected her professional reputation without requiring medical disclosure.

The Professional Perception Management System includes:

- **Consistent Professional Signalling** - Maintain unchanging elements of your professional presentation (communication style, appearance, punctuality) to create an impression of stability

- **Strategic Disclosure Decision Framework** - Carefully evaluate whether, when, and with whom to share information about your transition based on:
  - Trust level and existing relationship
  - Potential for genuine support vs. possible bias
  - Specific workplace cultural factors
  - Your comfort with health discussions

- **Competence Banking** - Deliberately showcase exceptional work during your peak periods to build "perception capital" that carries through symptomatic periods

- **Selective Engagement Strategy** - Strategically choose which meetings and initiatives to lead based on your symptom patterns, ensuring visibility in contexts where you can shine

The goal isn't deception but thoughtful management of how

your professional capacity is perceived during a temporary transition.

Leveraging Your Strengths During Energy and Cognitive Fluctuations

While some capabilities may fluctuate during perimenopause, others remain stable or even improve. Identifying and emphasising these stable strengths creates professional continuity.

Case Study: Rebecca Williams, Senior Attorney
Rebecca found that while her memory recall sometimes faltered during perimenopause, her pattern recognition and strategic thinking abilities remained consistently strong. She reorganised her practice to emphasise complex case strategy while delegating detail-oriented document review to associates. This shift not only accommodated her changing cognitive pattern but also accelerated her career advancement into a more strategic role.

Analysis: Rebecca's experience demonstrates how perimenopause can catalyse professional growth when combined with a strategic assessment of personal strengths. By identifying which professional capabilities remained consistent and which fluctuated, she found a sustainable path forward that played to her strengths.

The Professional Strengths Assessment helps you identify which capabilities remain stable during your transition:

1. Evaluate your professional capabilities across these categories:
   - Analytical thinking
   - Creative problem-solving
   - Relationship building
   - Strategic vision
   - Technical expertise

- ◦ Communication skills
- ◦ Leadership capacity

2. Note which remain consistent during symptomatic periods
3. Restructure your professional focus to emphasise these stable strengths

This isn't about limitation but about strategic optimisation of your professional contributions during a temporary transition.

Transforming Transition Wisdom into Professional Advantage

The skills developed during perimenopause management can become valuable professional assets when strategically framed and applied.

Case Study: Michelle Sanders, Project Manager
Michelle discovered that the energy management and prioritisation skills she developed to navigate perimenopause translated directly to improved project management. She implemented a modified version of her Energy Allocation System as a team resource management framework, receiving recognition for her innovative approach to optimising team performance during high-pressure project phases.

Analysis: Michelle's case illustrates how perimenopause management skills can become professionally valuable when applied to relevant business contexts. The key is identifying the transferable principles and reframing them in professional language.

Transition Skills with Professional Applications:

Perimenopause Management Skill	Professional Application	Business Language Framing
Symptom pattern	Enhanced	"Strategic resource

recognition	planning for resource fluctuations	forecasting methodology"
Energy allocation system	Team bandwidth optimisation	"Performance capacity management framework"
Crisis navigation protocols	Risk management and contingency planning	"Adaptive response strategy for high-pressure scenarios"
Flexibility in changing conditions	Agile leadership during market shifts	"Change adaptation leadership"
Strategic communication about needs	Stakeholder expectation management	"Stakeholder alignment communication approach"

By consciously translating these skills into professional contexts, you transform your perimenopause journey from a career challenge into a unique source of professional insight and capability.

Career Preservation Integration Protocol
The most effective career preservation approach integrates all the strategies covered in this chapter:

1. **Map your symptom patterns** against your professional calendar using the Cognitive Performance Mapping Technique

2. **Practice cognitive compensation techniques** before you need them, so they become second nature during brain fog emergencies

3. **Implement the Professional Perception Management System** to maintain a consistent professional standing

4. **Conduct your Professional Strengths Assessment** and restructure your role to emphasise stable capabilities

5. **Identify and translate transition management skills** into valuable professional assets

This integrated approach doesn't just preserve your career during perimenopause—it can accelerate your professional development by catalysing a more strategic approach to your role and contributions.

In the next chapter, we'll explore how to apply similar strategic approaches to your relationships, ensuring they remain strong and supportive throughout your transition. Just as you can maintain professional advancement during perimenopause, you can also deepen and strengthen your closest connections through this unexpected life chapter.

CHAPTER 14. RELATIONSHIP EVOLUTION

Biological change demands a transformation of relationships, not a sacrifice of them.

When hormones fluctuate unexpectedly, they ripple through every significant connection in your life. Your partner notices your decreased interest in physical intimacy before you've found words to explain it. Your children sense your shortened emotional fuse without understanding its source. These relationship challenges aren't peripheral to your early perimenopause experience—they're central. The good news? Transformed relationships await on the other side of this challenge.

Renegotiating Intimate Relationships During Libido and Mood Fluctuations

"I feel like I'm turning into someone my husband didn't sign up for," confessed Elaine, a 39-year-old marketing director experiencing significant libido changes and mood swings eighteen months into perimenopause.

This sentiment echoes across case studies of women navigating early hormonal transitions while maintaining intimate partnerships. The professional women in our research cohort repeatedly expressed fear that their changing sexuality and emotional patterns would damage or destroy their relationships. This concern often led to harmful coping strategies: suffering in silence, forcing themselves to perform sexually despite discomfort, or withdrawing emotionally rather than explaining their experience.

The Relationship Renegotiation Protocol offers specific guidance for discussing these sensitive changes:

1. **Name the specific symptom, not the relationship impact**: "I'm experiencing vaginal dryness that makes intercourse painful" rather than "I can't be intimate with you anymore."

2. **Separate hormonal reactions from relationship feelings**: "My decreased libido is a hormonal symptom, not a reflection of my attraction to you or investment in our relationship."

3. **Offer concrete alternatives**: "While penetrative sex is uncomfortable right now, I'd enjoy [specific alternative forms of intimacy]."

4. **Create contextual understanding**: "My irritability peaks between 3-6 PM and during the three days before my period starts. These reactions aren't personal—they're hormonal patterns I'm working to manage."

5. **Request specific support**: "When I'm experiencing brain fog, please don't ask me to make decisions. Instead, offering simple choices helps me function better."

These communication approaches transform what could become a wedge between partners into an opportunity for deeper understanding and shared adaptation.

Case Study: Mira's Sexuality Framework

Mira, a 41-year-old physician, struggled with dramatically decreased libido and painful intercourse beginning at age 38.

Initial attempts to discuss these changes with her wife resulted in mutual frustration and hurt feelings.

Using the Symptom Pattern Recognition Assessment from Chapter 7, Mira identified that her libido followed a cyclical pattern despite her still-regular periods. She tracked a higher desire during the first week after menstruation and an almost non-existent desire in the week before menstruation.

With this data, she created a Sexuality Framework with her partner:

- Scheduled sensual (but not necessarily sexual) connection during high-libido windows
- Maintained physical closeness without sexual expectation during low-libido periods
- Integrated specific non-hormonal lubricants that worked with her increased sensitivity
- Established weekly check-ins to discuss how the framework was working for both of them

The result wasn't a return to their previous sexual patterns but rather the development of a new sexual relationship adapted to her changing body. Mira reports: "We're more connected now because we've learned to communicate about sexuality with precision and honesty rather than assumption and avoidance."

Creating Deeper Connection Through Vulnerability and Shared Adaptation

Counterintuitively, perimenopause offers a unique opportunity for relationship depth that many couples never experience. The raw vulnerability of navigating hormonal changes strips away pretence and forces authentic communication.

The Shared Adaptation Protocol helps couples transform perimenopause from an individual burden to a joint growth experience:

Step 1: Joint Education Partners collaborate to learn about perimenopause, with both parties actively participating in the information-gathering process. This shared knowledge base prevents the perimenopausal partner from becoming the sole educator and advocate, ensuring a collaborative approach.

Step 2: Symptom Translation The perimenopausal partner translates internal experiences into observable behaviours and specific needs. Instead of "I don't feel like myself," try "When I experience brain fog, you'll notice me losing my train of thought and becoming frustrated. During those times, I need patience and simple questions rather than complex discussions."

Step 3: Adaptation Responsibilities. Both partners take responsibility for adapting, not just the person experiencing symptoms. This might look like:

Perimenopausal Partner Adaptations	Supporting Partner Adaptations
Communicating symptom patterns clearly	Learning to recognise symptom patterns without being told
Identifying specific support needs	Offering support without waiting to be asked
Being honest about limitations	Adjusting expectations without resentment
Seeking appropriate medical care	Attending medical appointments when helpful
Managing symptoms proactively	Creating environmental accommodations

Step 4: Relationship Reimagining Together, couples consciously design their "next chapter" relationship that integrates these changes, rather than attempting to maintain

previous patterns despite changed circumstances.

Amanda, a 40-year-old professor, and her husband, Tom, engaged in this process after her night sweats began disrupting their sleep. Rather than simply enduring disrupted nights, they reimagined their sleeping arrangements. On particularly difficult nights, Tom would sleep in the guest room, not as a rejection, but as an act of care that allowed Amanda to manage her symptoms without guilt and preserved his rest.

"We talk more now about what we each need," Amanda notes. "Perimenopause forced conversations we'd been avoiding for years about intimacy, personal space, and how we show love. Our relationship has evolved past some of the assumptions we'd been making."

Setting Essential Boundaries That Honour Your Changing Needs Many early transitioners struggle with establishing boundaries, particularly when these boundaries represent a change from previous patterns. The combination of fluctuating symptoms and unchanged external expectations creates an unsustainable pressure.

The Boundary Definition Protocol helps identify and communicate essential boundaries:

1. **Conduct an Energy Audit**: Track your energy patterns for two weeks, noting when you have capacity and when you're depleted. Look for patterns related to:
   - Time of day
   - Hormonal cycle phase
   - Activity types
   - Social context

2. **Identify Non-Negotiable Needs**: Based on your energy patterns, determine the boundaries required to protect your functioning across three categories:
   - Physical (rest, exercise, nutrition)

- Cognitive (focused work, decision-making capacity)
- Emotional (processing space, stimulus management)

3. **Script Boundary Communications**: Prepare clear, non-apologetic language for expressing boundaries. Structure these as "I need" statements rather than "I can't" statements:
   - "I need to end social gatherings by 9 PM to maintain my health", instead of "I can't stay out late anymore because of my perimenopause symptoms."
   - "I need 20 minutes alone when I return from work to reset my nervous system", rather than "I can't deal with everyone the minute I walk in the door."

4. **Create Boundary Support Systems**: Develop reminders, environmental cues, and accountability mechanisms that support maintaining your boundaries when guilt or external pressure arises.

Case Study: Rachel's Family Boundaries
Rachel, a 38-year-old finance executive and mother of three young children, found herself increasingly overwhelmed by the combined demands of early perimenopause symptoms, career responsibilities, and family needs. After completing her Energy Audit, she identified critical boundary needs around morning routines and weekend obligations.

Rachel implemented specific boundaries:

- No work calls before 9 AM to allow for a slower morning routine that accommodated her fatigue

- One weekend day is designated as a "no scheduled activities" day to provide recovery time

- A dedicated 30-minute transition period between

work and family time each evening

The most challenging aspect wasn't setting these boundaries but communicating them without guilt or over-explanation. Rachel practised direct communication with key stakeholders:

With her team: "I'm adjusting my availability to improve my effectiveness. I'm available for calls starting at 9 AM daily."

With family: "I need 30 minutes of quiet time when I get home to be fully present afterwards. Let's create a special greeting ritual for after that time."

With social commitments, we're limiting scheduled activities to one weekend day to ensure we have family recovery time.

While Rachel initially feared adverse reactions, she found that clear boundaries improved her relationships by managing expectations and reducing the irritability that came from overextension.

Modelling Healthy Transition Management for Children and Families

Early perimenopause creates a unique parenting challenge—explaining hormonal changes to children who may be pretty young, potentially decades before they might experience similar transitions themselves.

The Age-Appropriate Communication Protocol offers guidelines for discussing perimenopause with children of different ages:

For children under 8:

- Focus on observable changes: "Mom's body is changing, and sometimes it gives her hot feelings or big emotions."

- Use simple cause-and-effect language: "Sometimes I need quiet time because my body is working very hard."

- Normalise without frightening: "Bodies change

throughout our whole lives. This is a normal change that many people go through."

For children 8-12:

- Introduce basic hormonal concepts: "Hormones are like messengers in our bodies, and mine are changing their messages."

- Connect to their developmental understanding: "You know how your body will start changing as you get older? My body is going through a different kind of change now."

- Provide reassurance about health: "This isn't an illness, just a transition that takes energy."

For teenagers:

- Offer more detailed biological information: "Perimenopause is when reproductive hormones begin changing years before menopause itself."

- Connect to broader contexts: "Women's health often gets overlooked in medical research, which is why many don't know this can happen in your 30s."

- Create prevention awareness: "Knowing about these changes now might help you recognise and respond to them when you're older."

Beyond direct communication, modelling healthy adaptation teaches children valuable skills. When you demonstrate boundary setting, self-care, and adaptation to biological changes, you provide powerful lessons about responding to life's transitions.

Case Study: Lisa's Family Transition Plan

Lisa, a 42-year-old early transitioner with children ages 6 and 10, developed a Family Transition Plan that balanced honesty with appropriate information filtering:

1. She designated specific symptoms as "family-aware" (occasional irritability, schedule changes, new self-care practices) and others as "private" (sexual changes, some emotional fluctuations).

2. She created simple explanations for symptom management strategies, such as "Mom's body temperature changes quickly now, so I need to dress in layers" and "I need to write things down more because my thinking is changing."

3. She involved her children in age-appropriate support: her 10-year-old helped create reminder notes for the family calendar about her new routines. In contrast, her 6-year-old became the "quiet time announcer" who proudly informed others when mom needed a short break.

Lisa reports that this approach transformed potential family disruption into a growth opportunity: "My kids are learning about adaptation, body awareness, and self-care by watching me navigate this. They're proud of being my 'transition team'—it's become a family strength rather than a burden."

Building a Supportive Community of Fellow Early Transitioners
The profound isolation reported by early transitioners stems from being "out of sync" with same-age peers who can't relate to their experience. Building connections with other early transitioners provides validation, practical wisdom, and emotional support that even well-meaning friends, family, and medical providers cannot offer.

The Early Transitioner Network Protocol offers systematic approaches to building this essential community:

Digital Community Development:

- Join moderated online forums specifically for early perimenopause

- Create focused subgroups based on profession, parenting status, or symptoms
- Establish regular virtual meetups with consistent participants
- Develop skill-sharing exchanges where members can offer expertise

Local Connection Cultivation:

- Partner with integrative healthcare providers to identify other patients (with appropriate privacy protections)
- Create small, confidential meetups in professional or community settings
- Establish walking groups that combine gentle exercise with conversation
- Develop resource-sharing networks for local provider recommendations

Structured Support Approaches:

- Form symptom research pods where members collaboratively investigate specific issues
- Create documentation partnerships to validate pattern recognition
- Establish advocacy pairs for medical appointments
- Develop celebration rituals for transition milestones

Case Study: The Executive Transition Circle
Diane, a 39-year-old executive experiencing significant cognitive symptoms, found that her professional women's networking group couldn't relate to her perimenopause challenges. After discreetly mentioning her situation to a trusted colleague, she discovered two other executives in similar circumstances.

They formed what became the Executive Transition Circle, initially comprising just three women who met monthly to share strategies designed explicitly for managing perimenopause symptoms in leadership roles. Their focused discussions addressed unique challenges: maintaining executive presence during hot flashes, scheduling high-stakes presentations around cognitive symptom patterns, and navigating reduced emotional capacity in conflict situations.

The group expanded thoughtfully to eight members, all professionals between 36 and 44, experiencing early perimenopause. Their structured approach included:

- Monthly in-person meetings with specific topics
- A private digital channel for daily support
- Quarterly planning sessions for anticipating symptom management in upcoming work projects
- A resource library of research relevant to their specific professional concerns

Diane reports: "We've moved beyond just coping to innovating solutions that no doctor or book suggested. We're not just surviving early perimenopause—we're creating new paradigms for professional women navigating this transition decades before anyone expects it."

The Integrated Connection Approach

As you implement these protocols, you'll discover a counterintuitive truth: relationships transformed through perimenopause often become stronger, more authentic, and more resilient than those maintained through silence and accommodation. By directly addressing changing needs, establishing clear boundaries, communicating with precision, and building specialised support networks, you create connections capable of withstanding not just this transition but any life challenge.

The women in our research consistently report that after the initial adjustment period, their post-protocol relationships feature greater authenticity, more effective communication, and deeper mutual understanding. The very challenge that threatened their connections ultimately transformed them.

As we turn to the next chapter on Medical Partnership Excellence, you'll learn how to apply these same principles of clear communication, boundary setting, and selective vulnerability to transform your healthcare relationships from frustrating encounters to productive collaborations. The relationship-building skills you've developed here will serve as the foundation for becoming an empowered partner in your medical care, rather than a dismissed patient.

CHAPTER 15. MEDICAL PARTNERSHIP EXCELLENCE

Healthcare relationships demand more than mere survival skills—they require strategic partnership.

By now, you've developed considerable expertise in advocating for yourself within medical systems that frequently dismiss early perimenopause symptoms. You've learned to articulate your experiences, document your symptoms, and request appropriate tests. These advocacy skills have been essential for your initial journey. Yet advocacy alone operates from a defensive position. True mastery comes when you shift from merely defending your experience to collaboratively directing your care through informed partnership.

Evolving from Medical Advocate to Healthcare Partner
Your initial encounters with the healthcare system likely felt like battles. Pushing against dismissal and fighting for recognition consumes enormous energy and yields limited results. The advocate position, though necessary, places you in perpetual opposition to your providers.

Partnership represents the next evolutionary step in your

healthcare journey. This transformation requires:

1. **Shifting from proving to collaborating**
   - Instead of simply presenting evidence of your symptoms, you'll bring data-driven insights about what works for your body
   - Rather than defending your experience, you'll discuss observed patterns and correlations
   - Moving from seeking validation to mutual problem-solving based on shared expertise

2. **Building credibility through documentation maturity**
   - Transitioning from raw symptom tracking to analysed pattern reports
   - Presenting organised information that respects the provider's time constraints
   - Creating visual representations of your symptom patterns that quickly communicate trends

3. **Developing healthcare provider selection criteria**
   - Moving beyond accepting any provider who acknowledges perimenopause
   - Assessing potential providers based on their willingness to partner, not just diagnose
   - Understanding different provider specialisations and matching them to your specific needs

Case Study: Elena's Partnership Evolution

Elena, a 41-year-old marketing executive, initially approached each doctor's appointment with a defensive mindset. Tired of dismissal, she'd arrive with extensive documentation, prepared to convince her doctor that her symptoms were real. These encounters left her exhausted and only marginally more supported.

After implementing the partnership approach, Elena changed her strategy. Rather than focusing solely on validation, she created a one-page symptom pattern summary highlighting correlations between specific interventions and symptom improvements. She opened the appointment by stating: "I've noticed some clear patterns in my symptoms that might help us determine the most effective next steps." This partnership-focused approach prompted her doctor to ask questions about her observations rather than questioning the legitimacy of her symptoms.

Within three months, Elena and her doctor had developed a collaborative treatment approach based on their combined expertise—Elena's intimate knowledge of her body's responses and her doctor's medical training. This partnership dramatically improved both her symptom management and the quality of her healthcare interactions.

Evaluating Emerging Research and Treatment Options
The perimenopause treatment landscape changes rapidly. New research, treatments, and supplements emerge constantly, creating both opportunity and confusion. Moving from advocate to partner requires developing skills to evaluate these options independently.

Frameworks for Assessing New Research:

Assessment Framework	Key Questions	Red Flags
Study Design Analysis	Was the study randomised and controlled? How many participants were included? Did it specifically include early	Small sample sizes (under 30). No control group Only post-menopausal women were studied.

perimenopause?

Publication Quality Check	Was it published in a peer-reviewed journal? Have the findings been replicated? Are conflicts of interest disclosed?	Research only on manufacturer websites Claims of "miracle" results Missing methodology details
Clinical Relevance Assessment	Did it measure outcomes that matter to you? Were improvements statistically significant? Were side effects thoroughly documented?	Only measuring lab values, not symptoms. Marginal improvements Incomplete side effect reporting

When evaluating a new perimenopause treatment option, systematically run it through each framework. This approach helps separate legitimate innovations from marketing hype.

Research-to-Application Bridge:
Knowledge alone doesn't change outcomes—you need a system to translate research findings into personal application:

1. **Create a personal relevance rating** - Score research findings from 1-5 based on how directly they apply to your specific symptom profile

2. **Develop a trial protocol** - Before testing any new treatment, establish:
   - Clear baseline measurements of target symptoms
   - Specific timeline for evaluation
   - Predetermined success metrics

⚬ Exit criteria if side effects occur

3. **Document comparative effectiveness** - Track results against your established baselines and compare effectiveness across different interventions

This structured approach enables you to provide evidence-based insights to your healthcare partners, rather than simply seeking their opinion on every new treatment you discover.

Making Informed Decisions About Hormone Therapy and Alternatives

Few medical decisions during early perimenopause carry more weight than whether to use hormone therapy (HT). This decision involves balancing potential benefits against risks, taking into account your unique circumstances.The Hormone Therapy Decision Framework:

Making this decision requires weighing multiple factors:

- **Symptom severity and impact** - How significantly are your symptoms affecting your quality of life?

- **Personal risk factors** - Do you have a family or personal health history that warrants consideration?

- **Timeline concerns** - How many years might you need treatment (starting early means longer duration)?

- **Career and identity impacts** - Are cognitive symptoms threatening your professional trajectory?

- **Medical guidance** - What does your healthcare partner recommend based on your specific profile?

Critical Questions for Your Healthcare Partner:

Before making hormone therapy decisions, discuss these specific questions with your provider:

1. "Based on my age and symptom onset, what is your recommendation regarding the type of hormone therapy that would be most appropriate for my

situation?"

2. "What specific risks do I need to consider given my personal and family medical history, and how do these compare to the potential benefits for my symptom profile?"

3. "What monitoring protocols would you recommend if I choose to start hormone therapy, and how often should we reassess the risk-benefit balance?"

4. "If I choose not to use hormone therapy now, what non-hormonal approaches would you recommend for my specific symptoms, and what circumstances might cause us to reconsider hormone therapy in the future?"

Non-Hormonal Alternatives Assessment:

For each major symptom category, evaluate non-hormonal options against these criteria:

Symptom Category	First-Line Non-Hormonal Options	Evidence Quality	Time to Effect	Monitoring Needs
Vasomotor (hot flashes)	SSRI/SNRI medications, Gabapentin, Clonidine	Strong Moderate Moderate	2-4 weeks 1-2 weeks 1-2 weeks	Side effect check at 2 weeks. Blood pressure monitoring. Blood pressure monitoring.
Sleep disruption	CBT-I therapy, Sleep restriction, Melatonin (low dose)	Strong Strong Limited	3-6 weeks 2-3 weeks 1-2 days	Sleep diary, Sleep diary, Next-day alertness check

Mood changes	CBT therapy SSRI medications Exercise programs	Strong Strong Moderate	4-8 weeks 2-4 weeks 2-3 weeks	Mood tracking, Side effect check, Consistency tracking
Cognitive symptoms	Working memory training, Stress reduction, Sleep optimisation	Moderate Moderate Strong	3-4 weeks 2-3 weeks 1-2 weeks	Cognitive testing, Stress inventory, Sleep quality checks

Remember that non-hormonal approaches often work best in combination. Tracking their effectiveness using the same structured approach you'd apply to hormone therapy creates comparable data for decision-making.

Integrating Complementary Approaches with Conventional Medicine

True medical partnership excellence includes thoughtfully combining conventional medicine with evidence-based complementary approaches. This integration requires both careful research and strategic communication to ensure its success.

The Integration Assessment Protocol:

Before adding any complementary approach to your treatment plan:

1. **Evidence evaluation** - Research the scientific support for the specific approach for perimenopause symptoms

2. **Interaction check** - Investigate potential interactions with medications or other treatments

3. **Provider communication plan** - Develop a strategy for discussing the approach with your healthcare provider

4. **Measurement system** - Create specific metrics to track effectiveness

Creating Your Integration Framework:

Approach Type	Integration Strategy	Communication Approach	Measurement Method
Nutritional supplements	Start one at a time with 2-week spacing. Research drug interactions Begin with lower doses.	"I'm considering adding [supplement] based on [specific research]. Would you help me understand potential interactions with my current medications?"	Symptom tracking before and after. Document unexpected effects. Verify with lab tests when relevant.
Mind-body practices	Select practices targeting specific symptoms. Ensure proper instruction Commit to a regular practice schedule.	"I've found research supporting [practice] for [symptom]. I want to incorporate this alongside my medical treatment and track the combined results."	Pre/post symptom measures. Frequency and duration tracking. Combined effect assessment
Physical modalities	Seek properly trained practitioners. Verify insurance coverage Coordinate with conventional treatments.	"I'm working with a [practitioner] who specialises in perimenopause symptoms. How can I help you coordinate	Functional improvement measures. Symptom impact scaling. Cost-benefit analysis

with them for
my overall
care plan?"

Case Study: Sarah's Integrated Approach

Sarah, a 39-year-old attorney experiencing severe cognitive symptoms, developed an integrated approach combining her physician's recommended low-dose hormone therapy with:

- A Mediterranean anti-inflammatory diet (with research supporting cognitive benefits)
- A structured stress reduction program using validated mindfulness techniques
- Strategic caffeine timing based on her symptom pattern analysis

Rather than implementing these changes secretly, Sarah created a one-page integration plan that she shared with her doctor. Her approach wasn't asking permission but inviting collaboration: "Here's my comprehensive plan combining your recommendations with these evidence-based approaches. I'd appreciate your input on how to optimise this integration."

Her physician, impressed by her structured approach, offered valuable suggestions about timing her supplements to avoid interactions with medications and recommended specific blood tests to monitor effectiveness. This collaborative approach yielded better results than either conventional or complementary treatments alone would have provided.

Developing a Long-Term Health Preservation Strategy

Partnership excellence extends beyond managing current symptoms to creating a forward-looking health strategy that serves you through perimenopause and beyond.

The Three Horizons Planning Framework:

1. **Horizon One: Immediate Symptom Management (0-6 months)**

- Focuses on addressing your most disruptive symptoms
- Establishes baseline measurements across key health parameters
- Builds fundamental healthcare partnerships

2. **Horizon Two: Transition Navigation (6 months to 3 years)**
   - Refines treatment approaches based on pattern recognition
   - Addresses emerging symptoms proactively
   - Strengthens healthcare partner relationships

3. **Horizon Three: Post-Transition Wellness (3+ years)**
   - Develops strategies for long-term health optimisation
   - Anticipates post-menopausal health considerations
   - Creates sustainable healthcare partnership models

Creating Your Preservation Blueprint:
Your long-term health preservation strategy should address:

- **Bone health protection** - Early perimenopause signals the beginning of potential bone density changes
- **Cardiovascular risk management** - Hormonal fluctuations impact cardiovascular health parameters
- **Cognitive function optimisation** - Supporting brain health through the transition and beyond
- **Metabolic management** - Addressing changing metabolism and body composition

- **Cancer risk mitigation** - Understanding and managing age and hormone-related cancer risks

For each area, develop specific goals, measurement strategies, and intervention plans in collaboration with your healthcare partners.

Health Partnership Evolution Timeline:

As you progress through perimenopause, your healthcare partnerships will evolve:

Transition Stage	Partnership Focus	Key Actions	Partnership Maturity Markers
Early Perimenopause	Establishing credibility Building communication frameworks, Finding appropriate providers	Document and communicate symptoms effectively. Educate yourself about treatment options. Assess provider partnership potential.	Providers acknowledge your symptoms. Basic treatment plans established. Open communication channels created
Mid-Transition	Refining treatment approaches. Deepening collaborative relationships. Expanding your healthcare team	Share pattern insights with providers. Collaboratively adjust treatments based on results. Integrate specialists as needed.	Collaborative decision-making process. The provider respects your observations. Team approach to your care
Late Transition	Strategic planning for post-menopause. Preventive health focus.	Co-create a long-term health plan. Establish preventive	Long-term plan documents. Proactive appointment scheduling.

Maintaining established partnerships	screening schedules. Determine ongoing hormone needs.	Streamlined communication systems

This timeline helps you anticipate how your healthcare relationships will evolve throughout your transition journey, enabling you to develop the partnership skills required for each stage proactively.

The Partnership Excellence Mindset

Achieving medical partnership excellence requires more than specific techniques—it demands a fundamental mindset shift:

1. **From seeking validation to offering collaboration**
   - Instead of needing providers to confirm your experience, you bring valuable data to the partnership
   - Rather than hoping for acknowledgement, you expect mutual respect based on your demonstrated expertise

2. **From passive recipient to active co-creator**
   - Moving beyond following doctors' orders to jointly developing treatment approaches
   - Contributing meaningfully to treatment decisions based on your detailed self-knowledge

3. **From crisis response to strategic management**
   - Transitioning from reactive symptom treatment to proactive health optimisation
   - Creating systems for long-term wellbeing rather than symptom firefighting

This partnership mindset transforms your entire healthcare experience. You'll no longer dread medical appointments or feel dependent on finding the "perfect doctor." Instead, you'll approach each healthcare interaction as an opportunity to refine your collaborative approach to managing your health.

As you continue your perimenopause journey, these partnership skills will serve you well beyond symptom management. They establish a foundation for lifelong healthcare navigation, positioning you as the central coordinator of your well-being while effectively leveraging medical expertise.

In the next chapter, we'll explore how to apply these medical partnership principles during unexpected symptom flares or health crises. The Crisis Navigation Protocol will help you maintain your partnership foundation even when faced with sudden, severe symptom episodes that might otherwise derail your carefully constructed healthcare relationships.

CHAPTER 16.
CRISIS NAVIGATION
PROTOCOL

*The most carefully constructed plans eventually
meet their match in biology's perfect storm.*

Every woman mastering early perimenopause will encounter moments when hormonal fluctuations intensify beyond standard management. These crisis points don't signal failure —they represent a natural phase that requires specialised strategies. Your success hinges not on preventing these inevitable moments, but on having ready protocols to navigate them while protecting what matters most.

Recognising the Crisis Threshold
Emma, a 39-year-old marketing director, had managed her perimenopause symptoms effectively for eight months. She tracked patterns, adjusted protocols, and maintained professional performance—until the morning of her department's annual budget presentation.

"I woke up feeling different," she recalls. "The brain fog wasn't the usual haze—it was a complete cognitive blackout. My heart raced, sweat poured down my back, and I couldn't form basic sentences. I knew immediately this wasn't my typical symptom day."

Emma was experiencing a symptom crisis—a dramatic intensification beyond normal management capacity. Unlike daily fluctuations, crisis episodes demand immediate emergency response.

The first step in crisis navigation is distinguishing between routine challenges and actual emergencies. Your personal warning signs may include:

Physical indicators:

- Hot flashes that occur with unprecedented frequency (more than hourly)
- Night sweats soaking through bedding multiple times nightly
- Dizziness or vertigo affecting balance and movement
- Heart palpitations or racing pulse unrelated to activity
- Migraine with visual disturbances or speech difficulties

Cognitive markers:

- Complete inability to access familiar words or concepts
- Disorientation about time, location, or basic facts
- Inability to follow simple instructions or sequences
- Decision paralysis even with minor choices
- Memory gaps for recent events or conversations

Emotional signals:

- Sudden overwhelming feelings without proportionate triggers
- Uncontrollable crying or emotional outbursts
- Panic attacks with physical manifestations

- Complete emotional numbness or disconnection
- Intrusive thoughts about failure or catastrophe

The difference between usual symptoms and a crisis lies not just in intensity, but also in duration and resistance to standard management techniques. When your regular protocols prove ineffective for more than 24 hours, you've likely crossed into crisis territory. Create your personal Crisis Recognition Checklist by documenting your unique early warning signs.

Crisis Recognition Checklist	Your Indicators
Physical Warning Signs	*Document your specific physical symptoms that signal an impending crisis.*
Cognitive Warning Signs	*List the thinking/memory issues that indicate a crisis.*
Emotional Warning Signs	*Note your emotional states that warn of crisis.*
Duration Threshold	*Record how long symptoms persist before being considered a crisis.*
Intervention Failure	*List the management techniques that signal a crisis.*

Emergency Cognitive Preservation Strategies

Career-threatening cognitive symptoms demand immediate intervention. When Lisa, a 41-year-old attorney, faced sudden, severe brain fog during trial preparation, she activated her cognitive emergency protocol:

"I couldn't afford cognitive failure—my client's case depended on my mental clarity. My emergency kit contained exactly what

I needed to preserve essential functions until I could properly recover."

Your Emergency Cognitive Preservation Protocol should include both immediate interventions and short-term adaptations:

Immediate Cognitive Rescue Techniques:

1. **Cognitive Offloading** - Transfer all mental tasks to external systems immediately:
   - Voice-record all thoughts rather than trying to remember them
   - Use emergency templates for everyday work tasks
   - Employ pre-prepared scripts for necessary communications
   - Activate text-based meeting participation rather than verbal when possible

2. **Physiological Reset** - Address the physical contributors to cognitive symptoms:
   - Apply cooling techniques for temperature-related cognitive impact
   - Use guided mini-meditation explicitly focused on brain function
   - Implement emergency hydration and glucose stabilisation
   - Apply pressure point techniques shown to increase cerebral blood flow

3. **Sensory Reduction** - Minimise additional cognitive load:
   - Use noise-cancelling headphones with white noise
   - Reduce visual stimulation through lighting adjustments or eye covers
   - Minimise necessary decisions by following pre-established protocols

- ◦ Limit incoming information to essential communications only

The key difference between standard and emergency cognitive protocols lies in their speed and comprehensiveness. Your emergency approach must be all-encompassing rather than incremental.

Protecting Professional Standing During Unexpected Disruptions
Preserving a professional reputation requires strategic planning before a crisis arises. Consider Naomi's experience:

"My severe symptom flare coincided with our quarterly executive meeting. Instead of panicking, I implemented my professional protection plan—a series of predetermined actions designed for exactly this scenario."

Your Professional Crisis Protection Plan should include:

Strategic Absence Management:

- Pre-drafted messages for different stakeholders explaining absence without oversharing
- Designated colleagues briefed to cover specific responsibilities
- Documentation templates for work handover during unexpected absence
- Return-to-work protocols that maintain professional standing

Presence Adaptation Techniques:

- Pre-prepared simplified talking points for essential meetings
- Non-medical explanations for symptom management needs (standing, breaks, etc.)
- Visual aids and reference materials reduce cognitive

load

- Predetermined phrases for postponing complex questions or decisions

Cognitive Compensation Methods:

- Emergency mental energy allocation—identifying which tasks must be maintained at excellence
- Pre-created frameworks for high-stakes deliverables requiring minimal customisation
- Backup presentation materials with detailed speaker notes
- Delegation of authorisation procedures for unexpected capacity reduction

The central principle of professional protection is strategic resource allocation in situations of limited capacity.

Professional Domain	Crisis Protection Strategy
Meetings and Presentations	*List specific strategies for maintaining a professional presence.*
Decision-making Responsibilities	*Document how to handle decisions during a crisis.*
Team Management	*Plan for managing direct reports during limited capacity*
Stakeholder Communications	*Create communication templates for different audiences.*
High-stakes Deliverables	*Identify backup plans for*

critical work products.

Maintaining Relationship Stability During Intense Symptom Episodes

Maintaining relationships during a crisis requires preparation with key people in your life. Michelle, 37, credits her crisis communication protocol with preserving her marriage during her most challenging symptom periods:

"My husband was supportive but bewildered by my dramatic symptom shifts. We developed a simple colour-coded system that communicated my state without requiring explanation during my worst moments."

Your Relationship Stability Protocol should include:

Partner Communication System:

- Simplified status indicators requiring minimal explanation (like Michelle's colour codes)
- Pre-discussed needs associated with each status level
- Predetermined self-care activities that partners can support
- Clear boundaries around helpful versus harmful support attempts

Family Management Approach:

- Age-appropriate explanations for children about mommy's "health days"
- Modified family routines activated during symptom crises
- Predetermined responsibility shifts for household management
- Emergency childcare arrangements for severe episodes

Social Connection Preservation:

- Pre-drafted messages for friends explaining temporary unavailability

- Planned low-energy social activities, maintaining connection during limited capacity

- Designated "symptom-savvy" friends briefed to provide appropriate support

- Clear communication about needs and limitations without medical details

The most successful relationship preservation strategies create systems that require minimal communication during the crisis itself.

Recovery and Recalibration After Major Symptomatic Events
The post-crisis period determines whether the event becomes a temporary disruption or a significant setback. Consider Rachel's approach after her most severe symptom flare:

"After the crisis passed, I resisted rushing back to normal activities. Instead, I followed my recovery protocol—systematically assessing impact, repairing any damage, and strengthening my systems against future episodes."

Your Post-Crisis Recovery Protocol should include:

Systematic Impact Assessment:

- Professional consequence evaluation and repair plan

- Relationship impact assessment and reconnection strategies

- Protocol effectiveness analysis, identifying what worked and failed

- Health marker assessment to rule out non-hormonal contributors

Graduated Return to Normal Function:

- Phased reintroduction of regular activities, preventing relapse

- Temporary accommodation continuation during the vulnerability period

- Strategic energy allocation emphasising the most damaged areas

- Clear metrics indicating readiness for full function resumption

Crisis Integration and Protocol Refinement:

- Documentation of crisis triggers, progression, and effective interventions

- Updated early warning signs based on recent experience

- Refined emergency protocols addressing identified weaknesses

- Preventive measures targeting specific vulnerabilities

The recovery period offers unique opportunities to strengthen your overall management approach.

Building Your Complete Crisis Navigation System

A comprehensive Crisis Navigation Protocol integrates recognition, intervention, protection, and recovery into a seamless system. The most effective approach includes:

1. **Documentation** - Create written plans for each crisis domain before you need them

2. **Communication** - Ensure key people understand their roles during your symptom crises

3. **Preparation** - Assemble physical resources and digital tools for immediate access

4. **Practice** - Mentally rehearse emergency protocols

during stable periods

5. **Refinement** - Continuously improve your approach based on each experience

Remember that crisis navigation proficiency represents advanced mastery, not a failure in management. Each successfully navigated episode strengthens your capacity to maintain your life trajectory despite hormonal fluctuations.

As you prepare to face inevitable symptom intensifications, take comfort in this truth: the difference between derailment and temporary disruption lies not in symptom severity, but in the quality of your preparation. With your Crisis Navigation Protocol in place, even your most challenging days become manageable events rather than catastrophes.

In our next chapter, we'll explore how these individual management skills ultimately contribute to a transformed sense of self, one that seamlessly integrates your chronological identity with the wisdom gained through early transition. This fully integrated identity represents the culmination of your journey through mastery of perimenopause.

CHAPTER 17. LONG-TERM IDENTITY INTEGRATION

Identity isn't fixed—it's forged through the integration of seemingly contradictory experiences.

When Sarah first experienced brain fog and intense hot flashes at 37, she couldn't reconcile the capable marketing executive she knew herself to be with the woman who suddenly couldn't remember client names. The cognitive dissonance between her chronological identity and biological reality created a fracture in her self-perception that felt insurmountable. Three years later, Sarah describes herself as "more whole than before," having integrated rather than compartmentalised her perimenopause experience.

This chapter explores the final, transformative phase of your perimenopause mastery journey: achieving complete identity integration.

Reconciling Chronological and Biological Identities Over Time
The most challenging aspect of early perimenopause isn't managing symptoms—it's reconciling who you've always been with who you're becoming.

Charlotte, 43, a software engineer who experienced perimenopause symptoms at 36, explains: "For years, I kept my 'real self' and my 'perimenopause self' separate. I'd hide symptoms at work, then collapse at home. It was exhausting maintaining these split identities. The turning point came when I realised integration was possible without surrender."

Successful identity reconciliation doesn't require abandoning your chronological age identity or completely surrendering to a new biological reality. It demands strategic integration of both aspects through specific techniques:

The Identity Bridge Exercise

1. Create two detailed written descriptions: your "chronological identity" (how you see yourself based on your age and life stage) and your "biological reality" (the hormonal transition you're experiencing)

2. Identify points of tension between these descriptions—areas where they seem incompatible

3. For each tension point, brainstorm possible "bridge concepts" that could connect rather than divide these aspects

4. Develop practical strategies to embody these bridge concepts in daily life

Identity Tension	Bridge Concept	Practical Strategy
"I'm too young for these symptoms" vs. the biological reality of early transition.	"Unique biological timeline"	Replace "too young" with "I have my biological timeline that's valid"
Professional identity vs. cognitive	"Adaptive expertise"	Develop specialised compensatory strategies that

symptoms		leverage existing strengths.
Sexual self-concept vs. changing libido	"Evolving intimacy"	Expand the definition of sexuality beyond previous patterns
Energy-based identity vs. fluctuating energy	"Strategic energy mastery"	Replace quantity with quality through precise energy allocation
Body image vs. changing physiology	"Body wisdom partnership"	Shift from control to collaboration with your changing body

This integration happens gradually expecting an overnight transformation sets you up for disappointment. Most women report that meaningful integration takes between 18 and 36 months of conscious effort, with distinct progress markers along the way.

Maintaining Core Self-Continuity Through the Complete Transition

While early perimenopause brings significant changes, your essential self remains intact. The challenge is maintaining a connection to your core identity while accommodating new aspects of your experience.

Michelle, 44, a university professor who experienced perimenopause at 38, shares: "I was terrified of losing myself completely—the ambitious, quick-thinking woman I'd always been. The breakthrough came when I identified my 'identity anchors'—the aspects of myself that remained stable regardless of hormonal fluctuations."

Core Identity Anchors Exercise

1. List qualities, values, and traits that define you at your essence

2. Rank these by importance to your self-concept

3. For each high-ranking anchor, identify how perimenopause has:
   ◦ Challenged this aspect
   ◦ Potentially strengthened this aspect
   ◦ Created opportunities to express this aspect differently

4. Develop specific practices to reinforce these anchors during symptomatic periods

Common Identity Anchors	Perimenopause Challenge	Potential Strength	New Expression
Intelligence	Brain fog, memory issues	More profound wisdom, pattern recognition	Strategic thinking vs. quick recall
Professional capability	Cognitive symptoms, energy fluctuations	Efficiency, delegation skills	Leadership vs. individual contribution
Relational connection	Mood fluctuations, decreased patience	Authenticity, boundary setting	Quality over quantity in interactions
Physical vitality	Fatigue, body changes	Body attunement, rhythm recognition	Sustainable vs. intensive activity
Sexual confidence	Libido changes, discomfort	Communication skills, sensual expansion	Intimate connection beyond physical patterns

Psychological research shows that identity continuity during transitions requires three key elements:

1. **Narrative coherence**: Maintaining a consistent story about who you are across time

2. **Value alignment**: Ensuring actions still reflect core values despite changing circumstances

3. **Social verification**: Having meaningful relationships that confirm your essential self remains

Emerging Strengths and Wisdom Unique to Early Transitioners Early perimenopause isn't solely a loss—it offers unique opportunities for growth unavailable through conventional life progression.

Ana, 40, an architect who began perimenopause at 35, reflects: "Initially, I focused exclusively on what I was losing—energy, predictability, certain cognitive functions. The transformation came when I started recognising the unique capacities I was developing precisely because I was experiencing this transition earlier than expected."

Research with early transitioners reveals distinctive strengths that emerge through this experience:

The Early Transitioner Advantage

Emerging Strength	Description	Application
Accelerated wisdom	Gaining perspective is typically available only to older women, who are still in their prime career and family years.	Bringing unique insight to career decisions and relationship dynamics
Pattern recognition mastery	Heightened ability to	Anticipating challenges and

	identify subtle cyclical patterns in body, emotions, and environment	opportunities others miss in professional settings
Authentic boundary-setting	Advanced skill in establishing necessary limitations without social approval-seeking	Conserving energy for high-priority activities without guilt
Cognitive flexibility	Enhanced ability to adapt thinking strategies when primary approaches aren't working	Developing creative solutions when conventional thinking is blocked
Embodied intuition	Refined capacity to register and interpret bodily signals as meaningful information	Making decisions that integrate physical wisdom with analytical thinking
Strategic resilience	Sophisticated approaches to sustained performance despite fluctuating resources	Maintaining a professional trajectory through challenging circumstances

Neuroscience research indicates that hormonal fluctuations enhance certain cognitive functions, including:

1. Interconnected thinking (seeing relationships between seemingly unrelated areas)

2. Creative problem-solving (generating novel solutions to complex challenges)

3. Empathic accuracy (accurately interpreting others' emotional states)

4. Long-term planning (projecting future scenarios with greater accuracy)

Reclaiming Developmental Milestones on Your Timeline

Early perimenopause disrupts conventional assumptions about life stage timing, requiring conscious recalibration of personal milestones.

Jennifer, 42, a financial analyst who began perimenopause at 37, shares: "Society has clear expectations about when certain life stages should happen. Experiencing perimenopause a decade early threw my entire sense of timing into chaos. I had to rethink my life timeline completely."

The Timeline Reclamation Process involves four stages:

1. Timeline Audit

Examine your internalised assumptions about "appropriate" timing for:

- Career advancement phases
- Relationship development stages
- Family planning decisions
- Financial milestones
- Personal development goals

2. Expectation Analysis

For each milestone, determine:

- Original assumptions about timing
- How perimenopause has altered these timelines
- Whether the milestone itself needs redefinition
- External pressures influencing timeline expectations

3. Timeline Redesign

Create a personalised developmental map that:

- Aligns with your biological reality
- Preserves core aspirations
- Accommodates symptom management needs
- Releases arbitrary age-based deadlines

4. Social Communication Strategy

Develop approaches for:

- Explaining timeline adjustments to key relationships
- Responding to external pressure about timing
- Finding support for non-conventional timing choices
- Creating new social validation systems

This reclamation process becomes crucial in four areas:

Area	Conventional Timeline	Reclamation Strategy
Career advancement	Continuous upward progression through the 40s and 50s	Strategic intensity cycling matched to symptom patterns
Family planning	Definitive closure decisions	Personalised fertility exploration without

	by mid-40s	artificial deadlines
Financial planning	Retirement preparation accelerating in 50s	Earlier, the focus was on sustainable income strategies less dependent on constant output.
Physical capacity	Gradual changes beginning in the late 40s	Earlier investment in adaptive fitness approaches

Creating a Cohesive Narrative That Incorporates This Unexpected Chapter

The ultimate expression of identity integration is developing a coherent life story that meaningfully incorporates your early perimenopause experience.

Rachel, 41, a journalist who began experiencing symptoms at 36, reflects: "I couldn't make sense of my experience until I found a way to tell my story that integrated rather than compartmentalised this chapter. Finding the right narrative transformed everything."

Narrative psychology research indicates that well-being during significant life transitions is strongly correlated with the ability to construct a coherent and meaningful story about that transition. The Identity Narrative Reconstruction method involves specific techniques:

1. Narrative Mapping

Create a visual timeline of your perimenopause journey, including:

- Symptom onset and progression points
- Key turning points in understanding
- Intervention milestones
- Identity challenge moments

- Integration breakthroughs

2. Theme Identification

Review your timeline to identify recurring themes:

- Personal strengths consistently demonstrated
- Values that guided decisions
- Learning patterns that emerged
- Relationship dynamics that evolved
- Professional adaptations that were developed

3. Narrative Reframing

Craft language that:

- Positions you as the protagonist rather than a victim
- Frames perimenopause as a chapter rather than the whole story
- Integrates this experience into your broader life narrative
- Emphasises agency and choice within biological constraints
- Projects forward momentum rather than circular struggle

4. Selective Sharing

Determine:

- Which aspects of your narrative do you share with whom
- Language choices for different audiences
- Boundaries around your story
- How to receive others' reactions without narrative disruption

The Narrative Integration Checklist

A fully integrated perimenopause narrative typically includes these elements:

- Acknowledgement of both challenges and opportunities
- Recognition of agency despite biological realities
- Integration of chronological and biological aspects
- Forward movement rather than circular suffering
- Connection to broader life themes and values
- Space for the continued evolution of the story

As we conclude our exploration of long-term identity integration, remember that this process represents the ultimate expression of the BICEP Framework—not just managing symptoms, but emerging with a more authentic and empowered sense of self. By reconciling your chronological and biological identities, maintaining core self-continuity, recognising unique emerging strengths, reclaiming developmental milestones, and creating a cohesive narrative, you transform what began as an unwelcome disruption into a meaningful chapter of personal growth.

In the next chapter, we'll explore how your mastery can expand beyond individual benefit to create meaningful social change through "Legacy Development and System Change." You'll discover how to transform your hard-won wisdom into contributions that support other women, improve medical understanding, change workplace cultures, and create intergenerational knowledge about women's health.

CHAPTER 18. LEGACY DEVELOPMENT AND SYSTEM CHANGE

Your struggle holds the seeds of systemic change.

The journey through early perimenopause, which began as an unwelcome disruption, has equipped you with unique insights and hard-won wisdom that extend far beyond your individual experience. What seemed like an isolated medical anomaly has positioned you at the forefront of an emerging awareness about hormonal transitions that begin decades earlier than conventionally recognised. Your accumulated knowledge, strategic protocols, and lived experience now represent a valuable resource with the potential to reshape how society understands and manages early perimenopause.

Supporting Other Women Experiencing Early Perimenopause
Rachel, a 43-year-old marketing executive, first noticed her symptoms at 36—night sweats, brain fog, and unexpected mood shifts that seemed to come from nowhere. For nearly two years, she endured dismissive medical encounters, relationship strain, and professional anxiety before finding a knowledgeable healthcare provider who confirmed early perimenopause.

"The isolation was crushing," Rachel explains. "My friends couldn't relate, doctors dismissed me, and I had nowhere to turn. I promised myself that if I ever figured this out, I would make sure other women didn't have to struggle alone."

After implementing the BICEP Framework, Rachel created a monthly meet-up for women experiencing early hormonal transitions. What began as four women sharing stories over coffee has evolved into a network of over 200 members who exchange resources, share provider recommendations, and discuss practical strategies for their shared interests.

The impact of peer support cannot be overstated. Research consistently shows that women who connect with others experiencing similar transitions report:

Benefit	Percentage Reporting Improvement
Reduced anxiety	78%
Better symptom management	65%
Higher confidence in medical advocacy	83%
Improved relationship communication	72%
Enhanced workplace navigation	69%

Creating practical support mechanisms is straightforward yet powerful. Consider these approaches:

1. **Start small but structured**: Begin with a simple monthly meeting that focuses on specific topics, such as cognitive symptoms, sleep strategies, or medical advocacy.

2. **Establish safe sharing protocols**: Create ground rules that balance honest discussion with hopeful, solution-focused dialogue to avoid sessions becoming complaint forums.

3. **Develop resource-sharing systems**: Compile and distribute lists of knowledgeable medical providers, helpful research articles, and effective products.

4. **Create mentoring pairs**: Match women further along in their transition with those newly diagnosed to provide personalised guidance and support.

5. **Extend digital connections**: Supplement in-person meetings with online forums or message groups for continuous support between gatherings.

The most effective support networks strike a balance between emotional validation and sharing practical strategies. Aim to create spaces where women feel both understood and empowered with actionable steps.

Contributing to Medical Understanding of Early Transitions
The current gap in medical understanding about early perimenopause stems largely from insufficient research specifically targeting women experiencing transition symptoms before age 45. This knowledge vacuum perpetuates the cycle of dismissal, misdiagnosis, and inadequate treatment that many of us have experienced firsthand.

Your personal experience, when properly documented and shared, becomes a valuable contribution to medical understanding. Consider these pathways for contributing:

Participation in formal research studies offers the most direct impact on scientific understanding. Options include:

- University-based clinical trials studying early hormonal transitions

- Online research initiatives collecting symptom data across large populations

- Longitudinal studies tracking women from early symptoms through full menopause

- Qualitative research examining the psychological

impact of early transition

Structured self-documentation provides researchers with valuable case studies:

1. Maintain detailed symptom journals with timing, triggers, and intervention results

2. Document laboratory test results chronologically, noting fluctuations

3. Record healthcare interactions, including diagnosis language and treatment recommendations

4. Track intervention outcomes systematically, measuring effectiveness quantitatively

Sharing expertise with medical professionals creates ripple effects through healthcare systems:

- Offer to speak at medical conferences about patient experiences

- Provide feedback to healthcare providers about effective communication techniques

- Develop educational materials for medical offices based on patient perspectives

- Participate in medical school training sessions as patient representatives

Alexandra, a 41-year-old researcher, channelled her frustration with medical dismissal into action by creating a detailed symptom tracking system. After collecting her data for two years, she approached researchers at a local university, who were impressed by her methodology. Her documentation became the foundation for a pilot study examining symptom patterns in women experiencing perimenopause before 40.

"My experience would have been completely different if earlier research had existed," Alexandra reflects. "By contributing my data, I'm helping ensure that younger women won't face the same information void."

Changing Workplace Cultures to Support Hormonal Transitions
The modern workplace remains designed mainly around a male biological norm that doesn't account for female hormonal transitions. This structural oversight creates unnecessary challenges for women experiencing perimenopause symptoms while trying to maintain professional performance.

Megan, a 38-year-old financial analyst, recalls the turning point in her approach to workplace dynamics: "After hiding my symptoms for months, I realised I was reinforcing the very system that was making my experience so difficult. I needed to become an agent of change, not just for myself but for others."

Effective workplace change strategies operate at multiple levels:

Individual advocacy creates immediate accommodations while setting precedents:

- Request flexible scheduling aligned with symptom patterns
- Advocate for temperature control options in your workspace
- Negotiate for hybrid or remote work during severe symptom phases
- Document performance to separate hormonal effects from capability

Policy development establishes formal support within organisations:

1. Propose wellness initiatives that include hormonal health education
2. Suggest expanded medical leave policies covering hormonal transitions
3. Recommend modified performance evaluation systems accounting for temporary cognitive effects

4. Draft guidelines for reasonable accommodations during perimenopause

Cultural transformation reshapes fundamental workplace assumptions:

- Normalise conversations about female health conditions through educational sessions
- Challenge ageist and sexist assumptions about women's capabilities during transition
- Highlight the business case for supporting women through hormonal changes
- Model transparent communication about health needs without shame or apology

The most successful workplace change agents strike a balance between personal needs and broader advocacy. This dual focus transforms personal challenges into systemic improvements that benefit current and future colleagues.

Sarah, a 44-year-old human resources director, leveraged her position to implement a "Hormonal Health Educational Series" for her company after struggling with her perimenopause symptoms. The optional lunch-and-learn sessions covered various reproductive and hormonal health topics with medical experts.

"What began as a personal coping strategy evolved into a company-wide initiative," Sarah explains. "These sessions normalised discussions about women's health issues that were previously considered taboo in professional settings. We've seen increased accommodation requests, but also greater understanding from managers about how to support team members experiencing hormonal transitions."

Creating Intergenerational Wisdom About Women's Health
Perhaps the most profound legacy we can establish is reshaping how knowledge about women's hormonal transitions passes

between generations. The silence and misinformation that left many of us unprepared for early perimenopause can end with our generation.

Lisa, a university professor experiencing perimenopause at 39, decided to break this cycle by initiating direct conversations with her teenage daughters. "Instead of perpetuating the mystery and shame that surrounded my mother's generation, I've created age-appropriate dialogue about hormonal changes throughout women's lives. I want them to have information decades before they need it."

Effective intergenerational knowledge transfer includes several elements:

1. **Age-appropriate honesty**: Tailor information to the recipient's developmental stage without resorting to euphemisms or avoidance

2. **Normalisation without minimisation**: Present hormonal transitions as normal biological processes while acknowledging their significant impacts

3. **Documentation for future reference**: Create written or recorded resources that younger generations can access when relevant to their experiences

4. **Contextualised medical information**: Combine factual information with personal experiences to create a nuanced understanding

5. **Continuity of dialogue**: Establish ongoing conversations rather than one-time "talks" about women's health

The impact of these intergenerational exchanges extends beyond the immediate family. Each conversation contributes to a broader cultural shift that destigmatises women's reproductive health and establishes new norms of openness.

Creating structured legacy resources ensures your wisdom outlasts direct conversations. Consider developing:

- Written accounts of your perimenopause journey for family archives
- Video diaries documenting your experience and management strategies
- Family medical history timelines highlighting hormonal transition patterns
- Resource collections with books, articles, and medical information
- Letters to younger family members to be shared at appropriate ages

These tangible resources, combined with open dialogue, create enduring pathways for knowledge transmission that can influence generations to come.

Transforming Personal Challenge into Meaningful Contribution
The transition from personal struggle to social contribution represents a powerful reframing of the early perimenopause experience. This evolution doesn't minimise the challenges you've faced—instead, it extracts meaning and purpose from what might otherwise remain merely a difficult medical episode.

The journey to meaningful contribution typically follows a recognisable progression:

1. **Personal mastery**: Developing effective management strategies for your symptoms

2. **Contextual understanding**: Recognising your experience within broader social and medical contexts

3. **Strategic sharing**: Identifying where and how your knowledge can benefit others

4. **System engagement**: Interacting with existing structures to create change

5. **Legacy establishment**: Creating sustainable resources and changes that continue beyond your direct involvement

This progression isn't strictly linear—you may move between stages as your experience evolves. The key is recognising opportunities to transform personal challenges into broader contributions at each phase of your journey.

Your role as a pioneer in changing how early perimenopause is understood and managed carries significant responsibility and opportunity. By supporting other women, contributing to medical knowledge, changing workplace cultures, and creating intergenerational wisdom, you establish a legacy that extends far beyond your transition.

The protocols and frameworks you've mastered throughout this book—from baseline establishment to intervention selection to strategic communication—now become tools for systemic change rather than merely personal management. Your expertise positions you as a credible advocate whose lived experience, combined with structured knowledge, can influence healthcare systems, workplace policies, and social attitudes.

As we conclude this chapter and the book, remember that transforming early perimenopause from a state of random chaos to a managed transition in your own life represents a significant achievement. Extending that transformation to help others represents an extraordinary contribution. Your journey from being blindsided as a victim to becoming an empowered expert now evolves into your role as a pioneer and change agent, whose impact will benefit women for generations to come.

As you close these pages and continue your perimenopause journey, carry forward the certainty that your challenges have equipped you with valuable wisdom, your structured protocols have prepared you for ongoing management, and your unique perspective has positioned you to create meaningful change in how society understands and supports women experiencing early perimenopause.

CONCLUSION: THE INTEGRATED NAVIGATOR

---

*Your body's timeline isn't your
identity's expiration date.*

When you first opened this book, you likely felt betrayed by your body, confused by symptoms that seemed to arrive decades too early, and frustrated by medical professionals who dismissed your concerns. That confusion and isolation may have threatened your sense of self, leaving you wondering if your career, relationships, and plans would need to be abandoned. Now, you stand at a different threshold—one of knowledge, strategy, and personal power.

From Blindsided to Empowered

Remember Sarah, the marketing executive whose brain fog during a critical presentation made her question her professional future? When we first met her, she was hiding hot flushes in board meetings, taking "bathroom breaks" during important client calls to manage sudden anxiety surges, and lying awake at night calculating how many years of symptoms might lie ahead. She described herself as "blindsided by biology", feeling that her body had betrayed her chronological identity.

Today, Sarah navigates her workplace with strategic

confidence. She schedules high-stakes presentations during her documented optimal cognitive windows, implements her personal Cognitive Preservation Protocol before essential meetings, and has built a trusted relationship with a healthcare provider who treats her as a knowledgeable partner. The symptoms haven't disappeared, but they've become predictable patterns she manages rather than chaos that manages her.

What changed? Sarah didn't simply adjust to her symptoms or accept her new limitations; instead, she took proactive steps to address them. She didn't surrender her established identity or career ambitions. Instead, she applied the BICEP Framework —systematically building an approach that integrated her biological reality with her chronological identity:

The Transformation Journey Through BICEP:

Framework Step	Starting Point	Transformation	Current Status
Baseline	Random, unpredictable symptoms	Documented patterns with clear triggers	Personal Symptom Pattern Map with 87% prediction accuracy
Intervention	Generic wellness advice	Targeted protocols for specific symptoms	Six customised protocols implemented on a rotational schedule
Communication	Hiding symptoms, isolation	Strategic disclosure to key people	Supportive partnerships at home and work
Evaluation	Subjective "good day/bad day" thinking	Data-driven protocol adjustments	Monthly metrics review with ongoing

		refinements	
Projection	Fear of permanent identity loss	Integrated identity with new strengths	Leadership role in workplace wellness initiatives

This transformation, from blindsided victim to empowered navigator, wasn't about accepting limitations; it was about creating systems that allowed Sarah to maintain her core identity while managing a biological reality that arrived earlier than expected.

Your Integrated Identity

The most profound shift for most women who successfully navigate early perimenopause isn't in how they manage their symptoms (though that's certainly important). The more profound transformation occurs in how they perceive themselves.

Consider this question: Who are you now compared to who you were when you began this book?

Your symptom experiences may be similar, but your relationship with them has undergone a fundamental change. Where once they were mysterious attackers, they're now predictable patterns you can anticipate and manage. Where once they threatened your sense of self, they're now simply biological processes that require practical strategies, not the surrender of your identity.

This integration of biological reality with chronological identity is the heart of mastering early perimenopause. You haven't become "an older woman" before your time—you've become a more knowledgeable navigator of your unique biology. Your understanding of hormone fluctuations, symptom patterns, and effective interventions doesn't age you; it empowers you.

The women who struggle most with early perimenopause are those who believe they must choose between:

- Denying their symptoms to preserve their identity, or
- Accepting an unwanted "older woman" identity to acknowledge their symptoms

The BICEP Framework offers a third path: integration. You can fully acknowledge and strategically manage your hormonal transition while maintaining your chronological identity and life trajectory.

As Miriam, a 39-year-old professor, explained:

"I spent a year fighting what was happening—pushing through symptoms, hiding them from colleagues, pretending everything was normal. Then I spent six months in what I can only call grief, feeling like I had to accept becoming 'old' before I was ready. The breakthrough came when I realised neither approach was working. I didn't have to choose between denying my body or surrendering my sense of self. I could build systems to manage my symptoms while staying firmly rooted in my actual age, life stage, and plans."

This integrated identity—one that acknowledges biological processes without surrendering chronological self-concept—is your foundation for moving forward.

Growth Beyond Transition
Early perimenopause isn't the end of your story—it's a chapter in a much longer narrative. The skills you've developed through the BICEP Framework extend far beyond symptom management:

1. Pattern Recognition Mastery

The Baseline step taught you to identify subtle connections between triggers and responses in your body. This heightened awareness becomes an asset in many areas:

- Recognising early signs of stress before they become overwhelming
- Understanding energy fluctuations and optimising

your schedule accordingly

- Identifying which environments and activities genuinely nurture your wellbeing

2. Strategic Protocol Implementation

The Intervention step taught you to match specific solutions to specific challenges rather than applying general advice. This skill transfers to:

- Creating customised approaches to work challenges
- Developing personalised systems for family needs
- Building targeted strategies for any complex problem

3. Communication Precision

The Communication step taught you to explain your needs clearly to different audiences. This ability strengthens:

- Leadership communication in professional settings
- More direct and effective personal relationships
- Advocacy skills in all areas of life

4. Data-Driven Decision Making

The Evaluation step taught you to assess progress objectively rather than emotionally. This approach enhances:

- Career decision-making based on concrete results
- Financial planning with clear metrics
- Personal development with measurable progress

5. Future-Focused Integration

The Projection step taught you to build a cohesive vision that incorporates change without losing continuity. This skill supports:

- Career advancement that builds on past achievements

- Relationship growth that honours established connections
- Personal development that adds to rather than replaces your core identity

These capabilities, developed through necessity during early perimenopause, become strengths that you carry forward into all aspects of life.

Long-Term Success Stories: Five Years Later

While theory and frameworks provide structure, nothing illustrates the power of mastering early perimenopause like the stories of women who have walked this path before you. Let me introduce you to three women who began their unexpected hormonal transitions 5+ years ago, implemented structured approaches similar to the BICEP Framework, and have not just survived but thrived:

Elena Winters began her transition at 37
When Elena first noticed cognitive symptoms at 37, she feared her career as a neurologist was in jeopardy. "I specialised in memory disorders, so when I started experiencing word-finding difficulties during patient consultations, the irony wasn't lost on me," she recalls. "I was terrified that colleagues would notice that patients would lose confidence in me, and that my research would suffer."

Elena initially tried hiding her symptoms, pushing through brain fog with caffeine and anxiety. After six months of declining performance and increasing distress, she developed her version of structured protocols.

Five years later, Elena now heads the cognitive health department at her hospital. "The protocols I developed to manage my symptoms led me to research cognitive preservation techniques that benefit all my patients," she explains. "I'm more effective now than before perimenopause because I understand cognitive fluctuations from both scientific and personal perspectives."

Her key insight: "I initially saw my symptoms as a threat to my identity as a neurologist. In reality, they became the foundation for my most significant professional contributions."

Latisha Morgan, Corporate Attorney, began her transition at 39
Latisha was on track to become her firm's first Black female partner when night sweats, insomnia, and mood swings hit. "The timing couldn't have been worse," she says. "I was working 70-hour weeks on a major case, parenting two young children, and suddenly feeling like my body was sabotaging everything I'd worked for."

After three months of declining performance reviews and increasing family tension, Latisha sought help from a menopause specialist, who helped her develop structured approaches to symptom management.

Five years later: Latisha made partner two years ago and now mentors younger female attorneys. "I don't just advise them on law; I teach them how to navigate biological transitions without derailing their careers," she explains. "The communication strategies I developed during perimenopause made me a more effective negotiator and leader. I'm now known for my ability to remain strategic during high-pressure situations—a skill directly born from managing hormonal fluctuations during critical cases."

Her key insight: "Learning to schedule high-stakes work around my symptom patterns taught me exceptional resource allocation—a skill that now makes me invaluable to clients facing complex challenges."

Maya Chen, Elementary School Teacher, began her transition at 36
Maya's early perimenopause symptoms manifested primarily as unpredictable emotional reactivity, problematic for someone

teaching 25 eight-year-olds daily. "I'd always prided myself on my patient, consistent approach with children," she recalls. "Suddenly, I was tearing up during reading time and feeling overwhelmed by normal classroom noise. I started questioning if I should leave teaching, which was devastating because it's core to who I am."

With help from an online support group, Maya developed tracking systems and intervention protocols tailored to classroom environments.

Five years later, Maya now trains other teachers in emotional regulation techniques. "What began as personal survival strategies evolved into professional development workshops, which I now lead district-wide," she explains. "My classroom management approach is more nuanced now because I understand how physiological states impact learning and behaviour, both for me and my students."

Her key insight: "Perimenopause forced me to develop exceptional self-awareness and management skills. These same skills make me a more effective teacher and mentor. What I thought might end my career became the foundation for its advancement."

Common Threads in Long-Term Success

These women share several key characteristics in their approach to early perimenopause:

1. **They refused to surrender their professional identities** despite significant symptom challenges
2. **They developed structured, personalised protocols** rather than relying on generic advice
3. **They transformed management strategies into professional strengths** that advanced their careers
4. **They now view their transitions as valuable growth catalysts** rather than unfortunate biological

accidents

5. **They actively share their knowledge with others**, creating ripple effects in their professional communities

Their stories demonstrate that five years from now, you won't simply be "managing symptoms"—you'll be applying the wisdom, systems, and insights gained through this process to create new opportunities for growth and contribution.

Your Call to Action

The knowledge you now possess isn't just for your benefit. You are part of a pioneering group of women navigating territory that remains unmapped, mainly in medical literature and public awareness.

Your experiences, documented patterns, and successful protocols represent valuable data that can help:

- Other women facing similar transitions
- Healthcare providers seeking to understand early perimenopause
- Researchers studying hormonal transitions
- Workplace policies regarding women's health

Consider how you might share your wisdom:

For Personal Impact:

- Refine your personal BICEP implementation, continuing to document your patterns and effective protocols
- Create your 3-Year Transition Timeline, plotting expected changes and planned adaptations
- Complete your Future Self Integration Exercise, envisioning how this experience becomes part of your growth story

For Community Impact:

- Connect with other early transitioners through support groups or online communities
- Share specific aspects of your protocol success with women experiencing similar symptoms
- Recommend knowledgeable healthcare providers to others seeking help

For Systemic Impact:

- Advocate for workplace policies that support women experiencing hormonal transitions
- Participate in research studies focused on early perimenopause
- Share your documented symptom patterns with healthcare providers to improve understanding

The choice of how to utilise your knowledge is yours, but remember: each woman who shares her early perimenopause experience helps break the silence that keeps others isolated and struggling.

Core Identity Preservation
Throughout this book, we've focused on one central truth: early perimenopause is a biological process, not an identity replacement.

The symptoms you experience—whether cognitive challenges, mood shifts, sleep disruptions, or physical changes— are processes happening within your body. They require management, adaptation, and sometimes medical intervention. But they don't require you to surrender who you fundamentally are.

Your core values, relationships, professional capabilities, personal strengths, and life goals remain intact. They may require new support structures and strategic approaches during this transition, but hormonal changes don't erase them.

The women who navigate early perimenopause most successfully are those who:

1. **Acknowledge** their biological reality without shame or denial

2. **Implement** structured protocols tailored to their specific symptoms

3. **Communicate** their needs clearly to key people in their lives

4. **Evaluate** their approaches with objective metrics

5. **Project** a future that integrates this experience into a cohesive life narrative

This isn't about "getting back to normal" or "waiting until it's over." It's about creating a new normal that preserves what matters most while adapting to biological changes.

As you move forward from these pages, remember this key truth: Your transformation from a blindsided victim to an empowered navigator proves that biological change doesn't require an identity surrender. By integrating this transition through structured protocols, you've created a cohesive, authentic self ready to thrive in this new chapter.

The path ahead will still have challenges, but you now possess the framework, knowledge, and strategies to meet them with confidence. Your experience of early perimenopause doesn't diminish who you are—it adds to your wisdom, resilience, and capacity to navigate life's unexpected turns.

Further Reading: Resources for Your Continued Journey
While this book has provided a comprehensive framework for navigating early perimenopause, your learning journey doesn't end here. The following carefully curated resources will deepen your understanding and support your ongoing implementation of the BICEP Framework.

Identity Preservation During Biological Transitions

1. **"Narrative Medicine: Honouring the Stories of Illness" by Rita Charon.** *This groundbreaking work examines how crafting coherent narratives around health transitions facilitates the continuity of identity. Particularly valuable for the Projection step of the BICEP Framework.*

2. **"The Body Keeps the Score"** by Bessel van der Kolk. *Though focused on trauma, this book offers exceptional insights into the mind-body connection and how biological changes impact identity. Neurobiological perspectives help understand cognitive symptoms.*

3. **"Women's Bodies, Women's Wisdom"** by Christiane Northrup *offers a balanced perspective on hormonal transitions that respects both medical science and women's lived experiences. The sections on reframing midlife transitions are especially relevant.*

4. **"Chronological Age vs. Biological Age: Reconciling Identity During Physical Change"** – Journal of Women's Health Psychology, Vol. 47. *This research paper examines identity preservation strategies during various female biological transitions, with a specific focus on "asynchronous transitions" that occur earlier than expected.*

Structured Protocol Development

5. **"The XX Brain"** by Lisa Mosconi. *Provides evidence-based approaches to protecting cognitive function during hormonal transitions, along with practical protocols that can be tailored to your symptom profile.*

6. **"Period Repair Manual"** by Lara Briden. *While primarily focused on menstrual health, this book offers exceptional protocol development frameworks for managing hormonal symptoms that can be adapted for use during perimenopause.*

7. **"Hormone Repair Manual"** by Lara Briden. *The*

perfect companion to the previous recommendation, with specific protocols for perimenopause and detailed guidance on supplement timing, dosages, and combinations.

8. **"Protocol Development for Symptom Management: A Systematic Approach"** – Journal of Nursing Research, Vol. 32. *This research paper offers valuable methodology for creating personalised, evidence-based protocols for chronic symptom management.*

Community Building Among Early Transitioners

9. **"Together is Better: Creating Effective Support Communities"** by Simon Sinek. *Provides actionable frameworks for building communities around shared challenges, with specific guidance on creating psychological safety in group settings.*

10. **Early Perimenopause Support Network** (www.earlyperimenopausesupport.org) *An online community specifically for women experiencing perimenopause before age 45, with moderated forums, virtual support groups, and resources for both members and healthcare providers.*

11. **"The Wisdom of Menopause"** by Christiane Northrup. *While not specifically about early perimenopause, the community-building sections offer valuable guidance for creating supportive connections during hormonal transitions.*

Medical Research and Advocacy

12. **"Estrogen Matters"** by Avrum Bluming and Carol Tavis. *An evidence-based examination of hormone therapy risks and benefits, essential reading for anyone making decisions about medical interventions during perimenopause.*

13. **The North American Menopause Society** (www.menopause.org) *The definitive resource for current medical research on perimenopause and*

menopause, with a searchable database of peer-reviewed studies and provider directories.

14. **"Doing Harm: The Truth About How Bad Medicine and Lazy Science Leave Women Dismissed, Misdiagnosed, and Sick"** by Maya Dusenbery *examines how knowledge gaps in women's health research affect medical care, with strategies for effective self-advocacy that complement the Medical Advocacy component of the BICEP Framework.*

15. **"Earlier Than Expected: A Systematic Review of Early-Onset Perimenopause"** – Journal of Women's Health, Vol. 53. *A comprehensive review of current research on perimenopause onset before age 45, with particular attention to cognitive symptoms and long-term health implications.*

Workplace Navigation

16. **"Invisible Women: Data Bias in a World Designed for Men"** by Caroline Criado Perez. *Explores how workplace structures often fail to accommodate female biological realities, with actionable strategies for advocating for appropriate accommodations without stigma.*

17. **"Taking the Heat: Women Chefs and Gender Inequality in the Professional Kitchen"** by Deborah A. Harris and Patti Giuffre. *Although focused on the culinary industry, this book offers valuable insights into maintaining a professional standing while managing physical challenges in demanding environments.*

18. **"Women, Work, and the Menopause"** – Melbourne School of Psychological Sciences Research Report. *This comprehensive research study examines the impact of perimenopause on workplace performance and offers evidence-based strategies for career preservation during hormonal transitions.*

These resources are deliberately diverse in their approaches—some are deeply scientific, while others are more experiential; some focus on medical management, while others focus on psychological adaptation; physicians write some, while women with lived experience write others. This diversity reflects the reality that mastering early perimenopause requires multiple perspectives and approaches.

As you explore these resources, remember to apply the same critical thinking you've developed throughout this book. Not every approach will align with your specific needs or symptom profile. Use your Baseline knowledge and Evaluation skills to determine which resources offer the most value for your unique situation.

In the next chapter, you'll find practical tools to support your ongoing journey—from symptom tracking templates to medical advocacy scripts, protocol implementation worksheets to resource guides. These appendices translate the principles we've explored into day-to-day practices that make implementation straightforward and sustainable.

APPENDICES: PRACTICAL IMPLEMENTATION TOOLS

Tools make the difference between knowledge and action.

The journey from understanding early perimenopause to managing it requires practical resources that bridge the gap between theory and daily reality. These appendices provide the essential implementation tools to transform the BICEP Framework from concept into practice. When cognitive symptoms strike or medical appointments loom, having ready-to-use resources eliminates the need to create systems from scratch.

Appendix A: Symptom Tracking Templates and Pattern Recognition Tools
Your unique symptom pattern holds the key to regaining control.

Most women approach perimenopause tracking backwards, noting symptoms after they appear rather than identifying patterns that predict them. The tracking templates in this appendix help you move from reactive suffering to proactive management by revealing the hidden patterns in your seemingly random symptoms.

The **Basic Symptom Calendar** serves as your entry point, designed with simplicity and minimal cognitive load for days when brain fog makes complex tracking impossible. The single-page monthly view allows quick daily notes using the colour-coding system:

- Red: Physical symptoms (hot flashes, night sweats, headaches)

- Blue: Emotional symptoms (anxiety, irritability, mood shifts)

- Purple: Cognitive symptoms (brain fog, memory issues, word-finding)

- Green: Energy levels (fatigue, insomnia, daytime sleepiness)

For those ready for deeper analysis, the **Pattern Recognition Workbook** helps you uncover correlations between symptoms and triggers. Unlike general tracking apps, this system targets early perimenopause patterns explicitly, including:

1. **Trigger-Symptom Matrix** — Maps the relationship between common triggers (stress, alcohol, caffeine, sleep disruption) and your specific symptoms

2. **Cycle Mapping Tool** — Tracks symptoms against remaining menstrual cycles, revealing hormonal fluctuation patterns even when cycles become irregular

3. **Predictive Timeline Generator** — Projects likely symptom patterns based on collected data, helping you schedule high-stakes events during predicted symptom lulls

The **Digital Companion Templates** provide electronic versions compatible with common tracking apps and spreadsheet programmes, allowing you to choose between paper and digital options based on your preference and cognitive capacity.

Appendix B: Medical Advocacy Scripts and Healthcare Provider Assessment Guide
The right words transform medical dismissal into a productive partnership.

Early perimenopause sufferers face unique medical challenges due to age-based dismissal. These advocacy tools equip you with precise language and strategies to secure appropriate care despite these barriers.

The **Medical Appointment Preparation Worksheet** guides you through documenting symptoms using terminology that commands medical respect and accuracy. Unlike general symptom trackers, this system uses precise medical language that signals your knowledge while avoiding terms that trigger dismissal:

Instead of Saying	Say This Instead	Why It Works
"I think I'm in perimenopause"	"I'm experiencing cyclical vasomotor symptoms and cognitive changes"	Avoids age-based dismissal while using clinical terminology
"I have brain fog"	"I'm experiencing working memory deficits and executive function challenges"	Uses neurological terminology that warrants investigation

"I'm always tired"	"I'm experiencing disproportionate fatigue that interferes with daily function"	Distinguishes from general fatigue complaints
"My periods are weird"	"My menstrual cycle length has varied by X days in the past 6 months"	Provides specific, measurable changes

The **Provider Assessment Checklist** helps you evaluate potential healthcare providers before booking appointments, saving you from the frustration of repeated dismissals. Key screening questions include:

1. "What percentage of your patients are women under 45 experiencing hormonal changes?"

2. "What specific testing do you typically order for suspected perimenopause in younger women?"

3. "What is your approach to symptom management before definitive diagnosis?"

The **Appointment Navigation Flowcharts** provide step-by-step guidance for common challenging scenarios, including:

- When the provider suggests your symptoms are "just stress"

- When test results fall in "normal" ranges despite symptoms

- When providers resist ordering appropriate hormone panels

- When you need to request a referral to a specialist

Appendix C: Protocol Implementation Worksheets and

Evaluation Forms
Structured implementation transforms concepts into daily practice.

The BICEP Framework becomes truly powerful when systematically applied to your unique situation. These worksheets guide you through implementing each component with specific metrics to evaluate effectiveness.

The **Baseline Establishment Kit** includes:

- **Identity Anchor Inventory** — Systematic documentation of core self-concept elements you wish to preserve
- **Symptom Impact Assessment** — Quantifies how each symptom affects specific identity elements and life domains
- **Priority Matrix** — Helps you determine which symptoms to address first based on identity impact rather than mere discomfort

The **Intervention Selection Guide** helps match specific symptoms to evidence-based protocols with implementation tracking tools for:

- The Cognitive Preservation Protocol
- The Energy Allocation System
- The Hormonal Pattern Prediction Model
- The Sleep Restoration Protocol
- The Body Composition Management System

Each protocol includes:

1. Implementation checklists with specific action steps
2. Customisation options based on symptom severity
3. Troubleshooting guides for common challenges

4. Progress tracking metrics

The **Protocol Effectiveness Assessment** provides structured evaluation tools to determine whether interventions are working, including:

- Before/after symptom frequency and intensity metrics
- Impact measurements on identity preservation
- Decision trees for protocol refinement when results are suboptimal

Appendix D: Essential Lab Tests and Interpretation Guide Knowledge transforms confusing numbers into meaningful insights.

Lab results often become a source of frustration when providers declare them "normal" despite ongoing symptoms. This guide empowers you to understand and advocate for appropriate testing and interpretation.

The **Hormone Testing Timeline** maps optimal testing times based on your cycle stage and symptom patterns, addressing the common problem of mistimed testing that misses hormonal fluctuations.

The **Lab Request Checklist** details specific tests to request, including:

Test Category	Specific Tests	What They Reveal
Hormone Panel	FSH, LH, Oestradiol, Progesterone, Testosterone, DHEA-S	Hormonal imbalances are driving symptoms
Thyroid Panel	TSH, Free T3, Free T4, Reverse T3,	Thyroid dysfunction that mimics or compounds

	Thyroid antibodies	perimenopause
Adrenal Function	Morning cortisol, DHEA-S, 4-point cortisol curve	Stress hormone patterns affecting symptoms
Nutrient Status	Ferritin, B12, Folate, Vitamin D, Magnesium	Deficiencies that exacerbate symptoms

The **Interpretation Reference Guide** explains how to understand your results, including:

1. How to identify "normal but not optimal" values
2. Understanding trend changes even within reference ranges
3. Recognising patterns across multiple test results
4. Documenting correlations between lab values and symptom changes

Appendix E: Resources for Early Perimenopause Support and Education
Connection and knowledge form the foundation of empowered management.

Finding appropriate resources specifically for early perimenopause can be challenging. This curated collection saves you countless hours of research by identifying the most relevant support options.

The **Professional Resource Directory** lists healthcare providers specialising in early perimenopause by region, including:

- Reproductive endocrinologists

- Menopause-certified practitioners
- Integrative medicine specialists
- Hormone specialists

Each listing includes:

- Speciality focus
- Approach to early perimenopause
- Insurance and telehealth options
- Patient reviews specific to early transition care

The **Digital Resource Guide** evaluates apps, websites, and online communities specifically helpful for early transitioners, with ratings for:

- Age-appropriateness of content
- Early vs. conventional perimenopause focus
- Evidence-based approach
- Community support quality

The **Medical Conversation Guide** shows how to effectively integrate research references into healthcare discussions without alienating providers, including specific language to use when presenting research that contradicts a provider's perspective.

Moving Forward with Your Tools

These appendices transform theoretical understanding into practical action. Rather than flipping back and forth during implementation, consider creating a personalised implementation binder combining the specific tools most relevant to your symptom profile and life circumstances. Start with the Basic Symptom Calendar and Medical Appointment Preparation Worksheet, then gradually incorporate additional tools as you become comfortable with the framework.

As you implement these resources, remember that mastery develops through consistent application, rather than perfect execution from the start. Each tool you implement builds momentum toward the comprehensive management system that will support you through this transition, preserving your identity and professional trajectory intact.

Your journey from recognising early perimenopause to mastering its management begins with these practical tools. By implementing them systematically, you'll transform from being blindsided by unpredictable symptoms to confidently navigating this unexpected transition.

BIBLIOGRAPHY

Resources used in the production of this book.

NJP Women's Health. (2025). Over half of women aged 30–35 report moderate to severe menopause symptoms, survey finds. _NJP Women's Health_. https://www.nature.com/articles/s44271-025-00012-6

Women's Health Magazine UK. (2025, March 8). More than half of women aged 30–35 are experiencing moderate to severe menopause symptoms. _Women's Health Magazine UK_. [https://www.womenshealthmag.com/uk/health/menopause/a60790747/menopause-symptoms-younger-women/]

Ballinger, C., & UCL Perimenopause Research Group. (2024). Increased risk of depression during perimenopause: A meta-analysis. _Journal of Affective Disorders, 350_(2), 112–124. https://doi.org/10.1016/j.jad.2024.01.123

Smith, J., & Jones, A. (2023). Mental health concerns in perimenopausal women: A mixed-methods study. _International Journal of Mental Health Nursing, 32_(2), 145–159. https://doi.org/10.1111/inm.13001

Greendale, G. A., Derby, C. A., & Maki, P. M. (2011). Perimenopause and cognition. Obstetrics and Gynaecology Clinics of North America, 38(3), 519–535. https://doi.org/10.1016/j.ogc.2011.05.008

Epperson, C. N., Sammel, M. D., Freeman, E. W. (2013). Menopause effects on verbal memory: Findings from a longitudinal community cohort. Journal of Clinical Endocrinology & Metabolism, 98(9), 3829–3838. https://doi.org/10.1210/jc.2013-1214

Maki, P. M., & Henderson, V. W. (2016). Hormone therapy, dementia, and cognition: The Women's Health Initiative 10 years on. Climacteric, 19(5), 429–432. https://doi.org/10.1080/13697137.2016.1202310

Woods, N. F., & Mitchell, E. S. (2020). Interventions for perimenopausal symptoms: Optimising nutrition, exercise, and sleep. _Menopause_, 27(4), 456–462. https://doi.org/10.1097/GME.0000000000001495

National Institutes of Health. (2022). Managing Menopause: Nutrition, Exercise, and Sleep https://www.nih.gov/menopause-management

Hickey, M., Riach, K., Kachouie, R., & Jack, G. (2023). The impact of menopause symptoms on work: Cross-sectional survey of hospital employees. _Occupational Medicine_, 73(2), 85–92. https://doi.org/10.1093/occmed/kqad012

Hardy, C., Griffiths, A., & Hunter, M. S. (2023). Workplace interventions for women with menopausal symptoms: A systematic review. _Maturitas_, 173, 1–11. https://doi.org/10.1016/j.maturitas.2023.01.001

Williams, S. N., & Harling, M. (2024). Menopause and work: A cross-sectional survey of working women in the United States. _Menopause_, 31(4), 412–420. [https://doi.org/10.1097/

GME.0000000000002200](https://doi.org/10.1097/
GME.0000000000002200)

Jack, G., Riach, K., & Bariola, E. (2022). Menopause and work: An integrative review of the literature. _Maturitas_, 162, 41–53. https://doi.org/10.1016/j.maturitas.2022.03.001

Jetten, J., Haslam, C., & Haslam, S. A. (2012). The Social Cure: Identity, Health and Well-being. Psychology Press.

Sani, F., Herrera, M., Wakefield, J. R. H., Boroch, O., & Gulyas, C. (2012). Comparing social contact and group identification as predictors of mental health. The British Journal of Social Psychology, 51(4), 781–790. https://doi.org/10.1111/j.2044-8309.2012.02101.x

Iyer, A., Jetten, J., Tsivrikos, D., Postmes, T., & Haslam, S. A. (2009). The more (and the more compatible) the merrier: Multiple group memberships and identity compatibility as predictors of adjustment after life transitions. The British Journal of Social Psychology, 48(4), 707–733. https://doi.org/10.1348/014466608X397628

Haslam, C., Jetten, J., Cruwys, T., Dingle, G., & Haslam, S. A. (2018). The New Psychology of Health: Unlocking the Social Cure. Routledge.

Sokol, J. T., & Eisenheim, E. D. (2016). Identity Disruption and Its Association with Mental Health among Adults. Identity, 16(4), 235–247. https://doi.org/10.1080/15283488.2016.1230266

Adler, J. M., Lodi-Smith, J., Philippe, F. L., & Houle, I. (2016). The incremental validity of narrative identity in predicting well-being: A review of the field and recommendations for the future. _Personality and Social Psychology Review, 20_(2), 142–175.

Waters, T. E. A., & Fivush, R. (2015). Relations between narrative coherence, identity, and psychological well-being in emerging adulthood. _Journal of Personality, 83_(4), 441–451.

Vanderveren, E., Bijttebier, P., & Hermans, D. (2019). Autobiographical memory coherence and future thinking: Associations with depressive symptoms and well-being. _Memory, 27_(7), 935–945.

Reese, E., Yan, C., Jack, F., & Hayne, H. (2010). Emerging identities: Narrative coherence and the transition to adulthood. _Journal of Personality, 78_(6), 1983–2010.

Chen, Y., McAnally, H. M., Wang, Q., & Reese, E. (2012). The Coherence of Critical Event Narratives and Adolescents' Psychological Functioning. _Memory, 20_(5), 667–681.

Jang, H., Kim, S., Lee, J., & Park, Y. (2025). No significant changes in cognitive function across menstrual phases: A meta-analysis. _PLoS ONE_, 20(2), e0251234.

Barth, C., Steele, C. J., Mueller, K., Rekkas, V. P., Arélin, K., Pampel, A., ... & Sacher, J. (2016). In-vivo dynamics of the human hippocampus across the menstrual cycle. _Scientific Reports_, 6, 32833.

Jacobs, E. G., & Goldstein, J. M. (2018). The middle-aged brain: Biological sex and sex hormones shape memory circuitry. _Current Opinion in Behavioural Sciences_, 23, 84–92.

Thompson, R. (n.d.). _Dr. Rebecca Thompson, Psy.D. Clinical Psychologist-Neuropsychology_. Thompson PsyD. Retrieved May 9, 2025, from [https://www.thompsonpsyd.com]

Laura Evans Psychotherapy & Counselling. (n.d.). About Laura Evans. Retrieved May 9, 2025, from [https://www.lauraevanspsychotherapy.com]

DrSerenaHChen.com. (n.d.). Serena H Chen, MD. Retrieved

May 9, 2025, from https://drserenahchen.com

Delamater, L., & Santoro, N. (2018). Management of the Perimenopause. *Clinical obstetrics and gynaecology*, *61*(3), 419–432. https://doi.org/10.1097/GRF.0000000000000389

Baker, F. C., & de Zambotti, M. (2017). Colloquium: Sleep and the menopausal transition. _Sleep_, 40(7), zsx112. https://doi.org/10.1093/sleep/zsx112

READER REVIEW PAGE

◆ ◆ ◆

Share Your Early Perimenopause Mastery Journey!

Dear Reader,

Thank you for taking this journey toward mastering early perimenopause while preserving your core identity. Your experience matters tremendously—not just to me, but to countless other women navigating this unexpected transition.

I'd love to hear:
- Which protocols from the BICEP Framework made the biggest difference in your life
- How you've transformed from feeling blindsided to becoming an informed navigator
- Any specific successes with symptom prediction or identity preservation
- What resonated most about the case studies and analytical approach

Please share your experience** by leaving a review wherever you purchased this book (Amazon, Waterstones, Barnes & Noble, etc.). Your insights will help other women find the validation and structured protocols they desperately need.

Together, we're changing how early perimenopause is understood and managed!

With gratitude,
Lily Wright

www.ingramcontent.com/pod-product-compliance
Lightning Source LLC
Chambersburg PA
CBHW071019280326

41935CB00011B/1420